Infection Prevention and Control

An understanding of the social sciences within infection prevention and control (IPC) is important for those working in health and social care. This new book, *Infection Prevention and Control: A Social Science Perspective* positions the specialty of IPC as more than a technical discipline concerned with microbes. It is about people and their behaviour in context and the book therefore explores a number of relevant social sciences and their relationship to IPC across different contexts and cultures. IPC is relevant to every person who works in, and accesses health care and it remains a global challenge. Exploring novel approaches and perspectives that expand our collective horizons in an ever changing and evolving IPC landscape therefore makes sense.

Key Features:

1. Offers new perspectives beyond the topic area of infection prevention and control, to push the frontiers of knowledge and to challenge the status quo.
2. Interprofessional in nature and relevant to all those involved in the provision of medicine, health, and social care irrespective of their roles.
3. Truly international in nature in that the chapters have been developed by a range of individuals from across the globe.

Infection Prevention and Control
Control
A Social Science Perspective

Edited by
Paul Elliott

RGN, EN(G), EN(MH), RNT, BSc, MA, PGCEA, FHEA
Senior Lecturer in Adult Nursing
School of Nursing, Midwifery and Social Work
Faculty of Medicine, Health and Social Care
Canterbury Christ Church University, Kent

Julie Storr

RGN, BN (Hons), MBA, MHS
Independent Infection Control Consultant
Past President, Infection Prevention Society
S3 Global/KS Healthcare Consulting

Annette Jeanes

RN, Dip N, Dip IC, MSc, PhD
Independent Infection Control Consultant

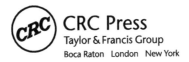

CRC Press
Taylor & Francis Group
Boca Raton   London   New York

CRC Press is an imprint of the
Taylor & Francis Group, an **informa** business

First edition published 2023
by CRC Press
6000 Broken Sound Parkway NW, Suite 300, Boca Raton, FL 33487–2742

and by CRC Press
4 Park Square, Milton Park, Abingdon, Oxon, OX14 4RN

CRC Press is an imprint of Taylor & Francis Group, LLC

© 2023 Taylor & Francis Group, LLC

ISBN: 978-1-032-45944-8 (hbk)
ISBN: 978-1-032-45838-0 (pbk)
ISBN: 978-1-003-37939-3 (ebk)

DOI: 10.1201/9781003379393

Typeset in Times
by Apex CoVantage, LLC

In Memory Of

Paul Elliott would like to offer a personal dedication to Noreen Crutchley.

I first met Noreen following my retirement from the Royal Air Force (RAF) in 1985, when she became my personal tutor whilst undertaking my conversion course from being an enrolled nurse to becoming a registered nurse at the Burton-on-Trent School of Nursing. Following this, Noreen and her husband, Wilf, became firm friends with my wife and me until her passing many years later. During the intervening years when initially being my personal tutor, Noreen was my guide, mentor and friend in helping and guiding me through what was a very difficult transition between the culture of the RAF and the culture of the National Health Service (NHS). There is no doubt in my mind that if Noreen had not been there, I would have floundered, and I feel without a doubt I would not be where I am today if it were not for Noreen. Following Noreen's retirement, we stayed in touch and visited on occasion, where she never ceased to advise and encourage me as a true and trusted friend.

Noreen, you always have a place in my heart and are held in my highest esteem and gratitude. In my mind I will always feel a sense of loss at your passing both as a colleague and as a friend. Noreen, you will be missed and are a great loss to the nursing profession.

Contents

Forewords

Working and teaching for many years in the field of Infection Prevention and Control (IPC), countless times I have heard that infection preventionists sometimes feel discouraged facing the daily challenges in health care facilities. Sometimes they get the feeling that things do not improve as much as necessary, no matter what they do. During the COVID-19 pandemic this situation was even more disheartening with the breaking down of the whole society and all the media pressure.

Definitely, the field of IPC is complex and goes much beyond the technical and microbiological perspectives. I am convinced about that since a long time ago, and therefore I was delighted by getting the opportunity to access this book. I can see it will be helpful for learning and thinking to develop a mindset that enhances our competencies to support better care.

Leonard Boff once wrote (1997) "the head thinks from where the feet step". Therefore, we need to recognize the social context in which people are in order to actually understand any situation. In that sense, this book is certainly an excellent source for reflections that can change the glasses that we are using to analyse the context of IPC and make positive changes in our actions.

When dealing day by day with IPC activities, it is of utmost importance to include both the health workers' perspectives and also that of the patients and their families. This book brings the concept of alignment between *compassion* and IPC, which I believe is vital to move forward and improve the outcomes of patients and families, putting IPC beyond the bounds of the biological approach.

I truly believe this book will inspire infection preventionists and all health workers and students who read it to make the change the world needs for safer and compassionate health care.

Maria Clara Padoveze
RN, MsC, PhD.
Senior Associate Professor, School of Nursing
University of São Paulo, Brazil

I am delighted to write the foreword to this refreshing and much needed book on the social and behavioural aspects of infection prevention and control. The theory and practice of infection prevention and control has generated many tomes that have been crucial in moving forward global ambitions to reduce the spread and impact of infection. This book signals a paradigm shift, with a focus on the role of people to complement the traditional focus on the role of microorganisms. It is particularly pleasing to see these authors – highly respected specialists in infection prevention and control – flying the flag for a holistic approach.

In my own work, as a researcher, practitioner and teacher of health psychology, I have collaborated with colleagues across the world who are trying to improve health. Never more than now have we needed to look at our health and care systems as composed of people; with all their own worries, roles, plans, intentions and habits. The threat of antimicrobial resistance is large, looming and, in some respects, already here with us. This threat alone should have us doubling our efforts to understand and drive behaviour change.

Perhaps the most refreshing thing of all is to see the focus in this book on kindness, compassion and understanding. It is too easy when discussing behaviours to fall into blame and judgement and for that to lead to interventions that are imposed on others. This book, in contrast, argues for us coming to a shared understanding, a shared motivation to improve and shared actions. This approach recognises the external forces that act on people and shape their behaviours and situates infection prevention and control within a complex system that acts on, and is affected by, every individual within it.

As a teacher of health professional students, I can see such value in starting here; in starting their learning in infection prevention and control with the human and then spreading out into the microbiological. The chapters are challenging and it is these challenges that will enable students to really reflect on their own practice as they enter the workforce. I would also encourage those whose roles are to lead others or to develop infection prevention and control strategies to read this book, hearing from other specialists about the practical advantages of understanding these social sciences.

The book covers many different and varied aspects of the specialty beyond the germs. As a researcher and practitioner, it certainly made me think. I hope that over the coming years we see more and more focus on the social sciences if we are to achieve sustained behavior change in infection prevention practices.

Lucie Byrne-Davis
BSc(Hons) MSc PhD CPsychol PFHEA FEHPS
Professor of Health Psychology
University of Manchester, UK

Preface

SOCIAL SCIENCE—THE BEATING HEART OF INFECTION PREVENTION AND CONTROL

A new book focused on infection prevention and control (IPC) and social sciences, written during a once-in-a-hundred-years global health emergency concerning an infection and the behaviour of human beings to stop its spread, could not have been timelier. With this in mind, there are two considerations that the authors want to highlight to the reader before they start to navigate the book. First, we strongly believe that an understanding of the concept of the social sciences and its implications within IPC is important for those working in health and social care. IPC is more than just a technical discipline concerned with microbes. It is about people and their behaviour in context. Therefore, it seems logical that the concepts underpinning some of the relevant social sciences are reflected in IPC approaches across all aspects of health and social care and across different contexts and cultures. This is worthy of exploration because IPC is itself relevant to every person who works in and accesses health care (Gilbert et al. 2014; Sutton et al. 2019), and it remains a global challenge in the fight against both emerging and re-emerging infections and the efforts to prevent their spread (De Vito et al. 2011; Warpeha et al. 2022). We are delighted to have the opportunity to expand our horizons and to look at an ever-changing and evolving IPC landscape against the backdrop of the social sciences. There is a growing appetite in IPC to look beyond the technical and towards the social, psychological and philosophical factors that influence human behaviour and consider these factors in an effort to strengthen the effectiveness of what we do in IPC. This is the ethos of the book.

We start by drawing attention to a previous book by Paul Elliott, *Infection Control: A Psychosocial Approach to Changing Practice*, published in 2009. This undoubtedly acted as a starting point for the current book. However, it is important to note that what you are about to read is for all intents and purposes a new book rather than strictly a second edition. In 2009, Paul explored the influence of psychology on behaviour change and practice improvement. We expand this thinking to a much broader consideration of IPC and the social sciences in all its diversity. We acknowledge that we probably still only touch the surface of many matters that comprise the social sciences.

Bajenescu (2021) identifies social science as a, "collective term for all those scientific disciplines that deal with the phenomena of people living together in society." However, bearing in mind that our world is made up of many differing races, cultures, religions and beliefs, social science can be reflective of societies that we, as individuals, do not have direct physical or social access to but may exist only in our imaginations. This can then impact upon beliefs and stereotypes or what we experience from sources such as the general media and, increasingly, social media, and this forms part of the underbelly of the book (Focused.Arts.Media.Education 2017).

The social sciences comprise a range of disciplines, including psychology, sociology, anthropology and philosophy—although there are many related disciplines that also fall into the definition (Kuper 2004). Throughout each chapter of the book, the authors address IPC-related issues related to the perspectives of different social science perspectives and disciplines. This may be subtle and nuanced or in some chapters up front and centre of what is being addressed. Each of the chapters offers a particular perspective related to IPC within a social science context and relates to the nature and behaviour of individuals and the influences that such behaviour has upon the individuals and environments.

There is of course a history to all this! Kousoulis and Tsoucalas (2017) identify a causal link between infection/contagion and society with regards to the transmission of the 1889 influenza epidemic from cities to towns and then villages with arguably people being the vectors (Martinus et al. 2020). Further, Villafruela et al. (2016) identify social interaction between individuals indicating a causal link between human-to-human socialisation and the transmission of disease (Bharti 2021).

Within this context you will see that the book has been divided into three distinct sections. Part 1 introduces in the broadest sense some of the theories and concepts that are picked up across many of the ensuing chapters. Given the expertise of the author, it reflects differing psychosocial and IPC perspectives within different contexts. The three chapters in Part 1 present an outline of a number of psychosocial theories and approaches and their potential relevance. In Chapter 2, Paul Elliott addresses the psychosocial nature of IPC and touches on matters of human rights and their relationship to safe IPC practices—a topic that is picked up in relation to both compassion and IPC leadership later. He also reflects on the myriad of influencers of the ability of practitioners to perform safely in the workplace, a theme that is explored in more detail by Helen Hughes in Chapter 6, Hugo Sax in Chapter 10, and Annette Jeanes in Chapter 16. The concept of truth and its relevance to IPC is the focus of Chapter 3, which also touches on philosophical aspects of the specialty, a subject revisited towards the end of the book by Julie Storr in Chapter 17. In his chapter, Paul Elliott also highlights the importance of being able to recognise alternative perspectives, including questioning the status quo, a point built upon across Part 2 of the book.

In Part 2, the focus is on leadership perspectives. Six perspectives are presented: leadership and influence; power and compliance; patient safety, governance and leadership; compassion, including both general issues around communicating with compassion and a specific angle on what happens in a compassion void. Part 2 concludes with an examination of why we do IPC at all! Part 2 reinforces the need for effective leadership and influence in IPC—including influencing at the highest level. Effective leadership has the potential to allow for an expansion of focus beyond the technical aspects of microbes and their transmission, towards the development of influential, powerful advocates capable of articulating and championing holistic, compassionate, people-centred care.

However, the chapter on power and the role of leadership in IPC in improving and supporting compliance takes thinking to a different dimension. The limitations of reliance on monitoring compliance rather than being visible and curious about what is happening are explored. Compliance and power are themes picked up in a number of chapters, including a novel take on compliance in Part 3, in which the language of compliance is itself explored, suggesting that even the word may be a problem. IPC is part of an overall approach to people's safety, and Helen Hughes explores the patient safety movement and how it has grown since the early 2000s. The important role of governance in safety is addressed. The chapter also outlines the need to take a systems approach to addressing the underlying causes of avoidable harm, including a focus on the people within the system and how best to influence their behaviour.

Compassion as a social construct (Blackstone 2009) is a permeating discourse within the field of healthcare quality (Fotaki 2015), and we are delighted to introduce communication and compassion as a stand-alone chapter, particularly since it addresses the service user perspective. A focus on compassionate health services, allows people's needs and values to be placed at the forefront of care, thus improving the overall quality of health services, and leadership is necessary at every level of the health system to stand as role model and embed a culture of quality. Insights are provided on what this means at the frontline through a clinician's experience with patients. Compassion and its relevance to IPC is emerging as a theme in recent times, so this chapter is a scene setter, introducing the reader to some of the concepts involved, the evidence and its application. To some this may seem to present an idealistic perspective—for example, where does compassion sit in the context of the facilities in which people work and constraints around capacity, human resources and access to medicines and technologies. These are valid considerations, but it is important to note that the chapter aims to stimulate the readers' interest in the topic and lay the foundations for subsequent IPC and compassion chapters.

Chapter 8, therefore, could be seen as applied compassion in IPC. This chapter uses the example of the restrictions imposed across health and social care during the COVID-19 pandemic and explores the adverse consequences associated with the restrictions and outlines the case for compassionate implementation of IPC guidance explaining how the two are not mutually exclusive. Part 2 concludes with a chapter on why we choose to work in IPC. Undertaking a role which aims to prevent a harm which may not be visible or evident can be difficult. This chapter outlines some of the reasons people choose to work in this area and the challenges they face. This includes reflections on motivation, role value and conflict, job satisfaction and being a specialist.

Part 3 then expands thinking to some real-world perspectives starting with a comprehensive exploration of human factors engineering in IPC. Human Factors Engineering is an interdisciplinary field of knowledge and practice based on engineering and social and life sciences and methods, to improve systems quality and performance. Hugo Sax presents a compelling case for its application in IPC but cautions that to realise this potential, healthcare institutions must allocate senior-level expertise and the necessary resources. Again—leadership comes into play. In listing a number of areas where human factors may play a beneficial contribution to IPC, Hugo Sax highlights the elimination of communication/guidelines ambiguity. In Chapter 11 Claire Kilpatrick probes the words used in the context of hand hygiene improvement as a case in point. This chapter explores the use of words and the meaning of language in IPC drawing on research that provides powerful insights into how the brain mediates behaviour, focused on mapping the semantic system, for example, the meaning of language within the brain. The chapter also considers the increasing application of social marketing in infection prevention and is testament to the value of communication in campaigning for change. A focus on the words used in an infection prevention context in the future could yield useful insights to support implementation of guidance into practice. Building on the campaigning theme, Chapter 12 turns conventional thinking on its head and presents the question of whether campaigns have unintended consequences and in fact make people anxious rather than reassured. Language is again a strong focus of scrutiny in this regard.

Social media is described as any media that facilitates social interaction, and its use has grown within IPC as a method of communicating information and influencing behaviour. In Chapter 13 we turn attention to the value it brings to the day-to-day work of IPC and consider some of the risks and unintended consequences particularly relating to the accuracy of the information that is put out via this media.

In Chapter 14 infectiousness and stigma in the context of HIV is explored with a focus on the narratives around HIV and AIDS that have dominated public health and IPC discourse for four decades. This chapter discusses the issues of stigma and infectiousness in relation to how gay men in particular have been impacted by HIV and AIDS. In Chapter 15 Pam Trangmar gives a very personal perspective of her role as a physician associate and her experience of aspiring to reduce the transmission of infection and maintain patient safety in the real world of health care. Her reflections on the reality of IPC in her area of work and her personal interpretation of what IPC means to her adds an interesting dimension to the book.

In Chapter 16 we return to some of the issues raised in the chapter on human factors, with Annette Jeanes focusing on IPC in the healthcare-built environment. Annette reflects on the role of IPC practitioners and the challenges in healthcare facility planning, design, delivery and operation—the complex interplay of people and organisations. It concentrates on psychological aspects of the healthcare-built environment in relation to IPC. It addresses the importance of collaboration and engagement between IPC practitioners and all those who work in health care, many of whom provide valuable insights on the day-to-day reality of the healthcare-built environment.

The book concludes with some musings on philosophy and IPC. The connection between IPC and philosophy has not received widespread attention outside of moral philosophy; therefore this chapter starts by considering IPC and the social sciences generally and looks back to some early work on anthropological aspects of IPC. Drawing on the limited literature in this area, the moral worth of microbes is explored with the conclusion that IPC has a value and a philosophical imperative to continue to do what it does to protect humans from harm.

What the reader will get from this book will be dependent on the background and the perspective of each reader. Health professionals will have different needs and expectations to a member of the public, for example. However, the book aims to offer a few learning objectives that provide the reader with the opportunity to do the following:

- Reflect upon a diverse range of perspectives beyond the purely technical and microbiological aspects of IPC, including and considering human behaviour and all of its influences with a focus on the psychosocial.
- Reflect upon how the diverse range of knowledge, expertise and experiences presented within the chapters of this book can offer opportunities to do things

differently or more effectively in the future, including influencing future theory and practice of IPC.

- Reflect upon your own knowledge, skills, attitudes, beliefs and stereotypes regarding IPC and how each can be enhanced by an expansion of thinking beyond the purely technical/biomedical (Ogden 2019) to a more humanistic/ social science understanding of IPC.

Paul Elliott, Julie Storr, Annette Jeanes
July 2022

Acknowledgements

We would like to acknowledge, thank and offer our appreciation to the following individuals for their help and support in the development of this book:

- We, the editors, would like to thank Shivangi Pramanik, senior editor, and Himani Dwivedi, editorial assistant at Taylor and Francis Group for their kindness, understanding and support regarding the time taken to complete the book during some very unexpected and trying times for all concerned.
- Paul Elliott would like to thank Jatinder Rangi, information technology lead support specialist, Medway Campus, Canterbury Christ Church University, for his advice and support.
- Julie Storr warmly thanks Jacq Cross for sharing her story in Chapter 8 and also acknowledges the stellar work of the campaigning groups: Care Home Relatives Scotland, Johns Campaign and Rights for Residents. She extends invaluable thanks to Dale Topley for his critical and philosophical review of Chapter 17.
- Hugo Sax warmly thanks Jonas Marschall, St Louis, for his critical review of Chapter 10.
- Thanks are extended from Claire Kilpatrik and Julie Storr to Martin Shovel and Martha Leyton of Creativity Works (https://creativityworks.net/), who were instrumental in shaping the work described in Chapter 11.

About the Editors

Paul Elliott commenced his initial nurse education in 1971 at Royal Air Force Hospital Ely, Cambridgeshire. Following this, Paul undertook a number of post qualification courses, including his aeromedical, specialist burns nursing and advanced resuscitation and clinical techniques, which enabled him to undertake a variety of duties culminating in a field nursing role attached to a tactical support helicopter squadron. Following retirement from the Royal Air Force in 1985, Paul entered the National Health Service, initially undertaking some further nurse education with the Burton upon Trent School of Nursing, Staffordshire. Following this he spent the next few years working in the accident and emergency/medical admissions settings before moving into higher education in 1991 with his current appointment being as a Senior Lecturer in Adult Nursing with Canterbury Christ Church University, Kent. Since entering higher education, Paul's primary research interests, publications and conference papers have centred around the psychosocial aspects of infection prevention and control.

Julie Storr is an MBA graduate and graduate nurse from the University of Manchester, where she also trained as a health visitor. She is cofounder and director at S3 Global and has worked internationally since 2005, predominantly as an expert with World Health Organization (WHO) on the development, implementation and evaluation of initiatives in the field of patient safety, quality and infection prevention and control (IPC). In recent years her portfolio has included work with WHO's Water Sanitation and Health (WASH) programme as well as IPC, Quality of Care and AMR. She led on the development of WHO's first IPC Guidelines and associated implementation packages. She was previously president of the Infection Prevention Society of the UK and Ireland, assistant director at the English National Patient Safety Agency and director of the award-winning national clean**your**hands™ campaign. She is an honorary advisor at Tropical Health Education Trust and a steering group member of Health Information For All (HIFA). Julie has published widely in peer-reviewed journals and is a regular speaker at international conferences. She was recently awarded a masters in health science from Johns Hopkins School of Public Health and is also a trained clinical hypnotherapist.

Annette Jeanes is an independent consultant infection control nurse. She was the infection control lead at the Nightingale Hospital in London for the duration of the initial and subsequent London COVID-19 response. Prior to that, Annette worked in the NHS as the director of infection prevention and control and consultant nurse infection control at University College London Hospitals. She has worked at several London hospitals in infection control, intensive care, infectious diseases, medicine and surgery. She has undertaken and published research in improving hand hygiene compliance and hospital cleaning.

Contributors

Nana Afriyie Mensah Abrampah, BSc, MSc
Advisor, UNOPS
Geneva, Switzerland

Louis Ako-Egbe, MD
District Health Manager
WHO Country Office
Liberia

Melissa Kleine-Bingham, RN, MPH
Technical Officer, Infection Prevention
    and Control
WHO Nepal

John Gilmore-Kavanagh, PhD, MSoc. Sc, Grad Dip, BSc, RGN, FHEA
Assistant Professor in Nursing
School of Nursing, Midwifery and
    Health Systems
University College
Dublin, Ireland

Sheila Hall, RGN, SCM, MSc
Retired

Helen Hughes, BSc, CIPFA
Chief Executive
Patient Safety Learning

Claire Kilpatrick, RN, PG Dip ICN, MSc, MFTM RCPS (Glas)
Consultant/Director
S3 Global

Hugo Sax, MD
Department of Infectious Diseases
    Bern University Hospital
University of Bern
Bern, Switzerland

Shamsuzzoha Babar Syed, MD MPH DPH(Cantab) FACPM
Head of Unit, Quality of Care
World Health Organization
Geneva

Pam Trangmar, MSc, PA-R
Deputy Course Director
Physician Associate Studies
Medway Campus
Canterbury Christ Church University

Note from the Editors

Although the contents of this book have been peer-reviewed, the thoughts and opinions are those of the specific chapter author(s) and may not reflect the thoughts of the editors. If you wish to offer any feedback relating to the content of any of the chapters, it is requested that you contact the individual author(s) directly.

REFERENCES

Bajenescu, T. (2021), Understanding the social sciences, *Journal of Social Sciences*, IV (4), 6–15.

Bharti, N. (2021), Linking human behaviors and infectious diseases, *Biological Sciences*, 118 (11), 1–3.

Blackstone, A. (2009), Doing good, being good, and the social construction of compassion, *Journal of Contemporary Ethnography*, 38 (1), 85–116.

De Vito, C., Marzuillo, C., D'Andrea, E., Romano, F. and Villari, P. (2011), Emerging and re-emerging infectious diseases: Tackling the challenge on a global level, *Italian Journal of Public Health*, 8 (1), 1–4.

Focused.Arts.Media.Education (2017), Microaggressions in the classroom, 15 May, Available Online at: www.youtube.com/watch?v=ZahtlxW2CIQ Accessed: 28 June 2022.

Fotaki, M. (2015), Why and how is compassion necessary to provide good quality healthcare? *International Journal of Health Policy and Management*, 4 (4), 199–201.

Gilbert, L., Iredell, J. and Merlino, J. (2014), Healthcare infection prevention and control really is everyone's business, *Microbiology Australia*, 35, 3–4.

Kousoulis, A. and Tsoucalas, G. (2017), Infection, contagion and causality in colonial Britain: The 1819–90 influenza pandemic and the British medical journal, *Le Infezioni in Medicina*, 3, 288–291.

Kuper, A. (2004), *The Social Science Encyclopedia*, Routledge.

Martinus, K., Pauli, N., Gunawardena, A. and Kragt, M. (2020), *Humans as Hosts, Vectors and Agents of Environmental Change*, The University of Western Australia, Perth, Western Australia.

Ogden, J. (2019), *Health Psychology*, London, McGraw Hill, 5–10.

Sutton, E., Brewster, L. and Tarrant, C. (2019), Making infection prevention and control everyone's business? Hospital staff views on patient involvement, *Health Expectations*, 22, 650–656.

Villafruela, J., Olmedo, I. and San José, J. (2016), Influence of human breathing modes on airborne cross infection risk, *Building and Environment*, 106, 340–351.

Warpeha, K., Chen, S. and Mullie, C. (2022), Editorial: Emerging infectious and vector-borne diseases: A global challenge, *Frontiers in Public Health*, Volume II, 10.

PART 1

Psychosocial Perspectives

Psychosocial Theories and Approaches

1

Their Impact Upon Infection Prevention and Control

Paul Elliott

Contents

DOI: 10.1201/9781003379393-2

1.1 INTRODUCTION

IPC has a long and varied history in terms of both the passage of time and current appropriate IPC practice. Yet despite both the quality of IPC, professional practice remains a challenge in terms of maintaining the safety of colleagues, those who seek health care, and all the interventions that accompany it. So the question that must be asked is why this should be the case in the twenty-first century, when a knowledge of sanitation, IPC and public health can be traced back to the time of ancient Rome (Karabatos et al. 2021). Sadly, with the fall of Rome, the rise of the dark ages and through the early modern era, becoming ill or contracting an infection was always a risk (Smith et al. 2012) until the work of Florence Nightingale (1820 to 1910), Ignaz Semmelweis (1818 to 1865), John Snow (1813 to 1858), Ernst Von Bergmann (1836 to 1907), William Halstead (1852 to 1922) and Joseph Lister (1827 to 1912) became known and was acted upon. Yet despite these and other advances in our knowledge of IPC, today a biomedical approach still appears to exert an influence on practice in the form of physically orientated behaviours despite the works of, for example, Creedon (2006), Elliott (2009), Williams (2012), Turabian (2018) and many more. Therefore, this chapter offers a flavour of the range of psychosocial theories and approaches that may be of relevance to IPC practice, summarised in diagram 1.1.

Each of these concepts are now summarised to offer an insight into their applicability to IPC and highlight the complex interplay of factors that influence human behaviour.

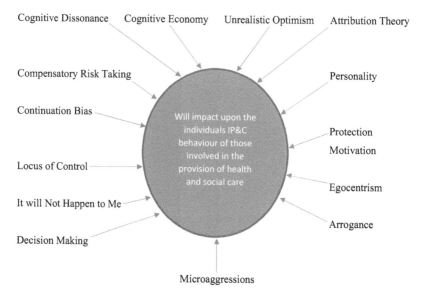

DIAGRAM 1.1 Psychosocial Theories and Concepts

1.2 COGNITIVE DISSONANCE

The concept of cognitive dissonance was originally identified by Festinger (1962), who proposed that, at a psychological level, the individual will strive to make consistent two or more things that would not naturally be so. In effect, dissonance is when an individual generates a reason to justify a previous behaviour or the undertaking of a future behaviour. Hand hygiene is an example, where the individual understands its importance in reducing transmission of infection but fails to perform it at the right time or in the correct way. Although hand hygiene compliance is influenced by multiple factors, from the cognitive dissonance perspective, it could be the case that to alleviate or reduce psychological conflict, health workers will establish a reason why, for example, they missed out part of the hand hygiene process or failed to dry their hands properly (Gammon and Hunt 2020). In general, dissonance has been perceived as serving to support behaviours. However, the findings of Chandu et al. (2022) suggest that although such a process has been argued to be problematic where behavioural change is concerned, by developing a situation where a discrepancy between what individuals know and how they practice may have positive effects upon future health-promoting behaviours. It remains to be determined whether or not such an approach to the application of dissonance could produce long-term health-promoting IPC behaviours.

1.3 COGNITIVE ECONOMY

In cognitive economy (Roth and Frisby 1992), an individual becomes tunnel-visioned, leading to context-specific task orientation not only in relation to their own behaviours but also their perception of what is occurring around them and will fail to consider the wider implications. Instead of being person-centred, the individual will become singularly focused towards achieving a goal or set of goals that will meet their own needs at the expense of ensuring their practice remains safe.

1.4 UNREALISTIC OPTIMISM

In unrealistic optimism (Weinstein 1982; Jefferson et al. 2017; Ogden 2019), an individual becomes unrealistically optimistic regarding risks. They may place themselves and others in what can be described as risky behaviour, which constitutes unsafe IPC practice. Unrealistic optimism can be facilitated through lack of personal experience (Welkenhuysen et al. 1996; Ogden 2019). An individual's failure to adopt safe IPC practice is often linked to two beliefs:

1. There is no perceived risk to themselves or the risk of transmission of infection to others is so insignificant that it simply does not matter.

2. Even if there is a risk, it will not involve them. That is, even if the individual involved does transfer microbes and contributes to the development of a HAI to others, they will rationalise that it was not their fault or they will not be found out and held responsible.

1.5 ATTRIBUTION THEORY

Attribution theory is related to how individuals make judgements about themselves and others' behaviour (Ayers and De Visser 2018). Ogden (2019) suggests that this theory reflects attributions of self (internal) as well as attributions of others (external). Individuals can be extremely good at applying attributions when things go wrong, but as Parker and Davies (2020) indicate, these attributions can be unjustly applied, particularly when the individual is attempting to protect their own ego-related attributions of self. However, such attributions may emanate from stereotypes consistent with discrimination, disability, religious prejudice, ageism, racism, gender reassignment or sexism. From an IPC perspective, internal attributions could lead to the individual believing a certain thing about their practice, which may be positive or negative in nature. External attributions are related to where individuals will offer judgements about others' IPC practice but may not perceive the same in themselves. For example, I believe my IPC practice is safe, but my superior criticises it because of personal biases such as they do not like me.

1.6 PERSONALITY

Personality can offer causal reasons as to why individuals do or do not adopt appropriate IPC practice within the context of the structure of personality. Diagram 1.2 illustrates this concept.

In this concept, the structure of personality consists of the id, the ego, and the superego (McLeod 2016). For illustration purposes, the following example focuses on the id and the superego. The individual who is task-orientated, unrealistically optimistic, and cognitively economic will have the propensity to practice within the context of the id (Siegfried 2014). That is, being self-orientated within the context of the pleasure principle (Barnhart 1972) being a driving force of the id, where the individual gains pleasure from completing their workload on time but fails to recognise that in doing such, they may have enhanced the potential for transmission of infection by taking shortcuts in their IPC practice. In contrast, the individual who is person-centred in their practice and recognises the importance of following policy and process will likely practice within the context of the superego. Such Freudian influences, while acknowledged from a historical perspective, are perhaps less important in modern psychosocial thinking.

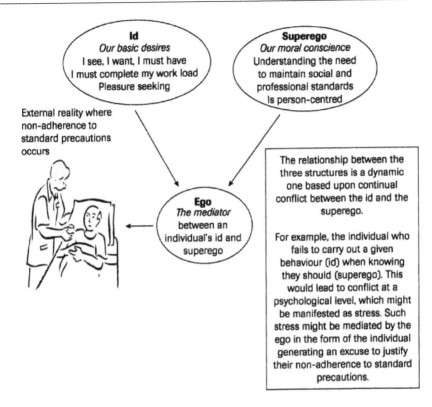

DIAGRAM 1.2   The Structure of Personality: Id, Ego, Superego

Source: (McLeod 2016)
(Freud in Slack 1981)

1.7 PROTECTION MOTIVATION

In health and social care, the pressures placed upon individuals in undertaking their roles and the challenges placed before them in an IPC context can result in individuals calculating risks to themselves. List 1.1 presents five elements of protection motivation related to IPC practices (Ogden 2019).

LIST 1.1 ELEMENTS OF PROTECTION MOTIVATION RELATED TO IPC PRACTICE

- **Severity:** The individual assesses the potential severity of retribution to themselves should they be identified as failing to adopt appropriate IPC practice according to the intervention they are about to undertake.

- **Susceptibility:** The individual assesses the potential for being identified if they fail to adopt appropriate IPC practice when undertaking a particular intervention where IPC would be a necessary requirement.
- **Responsive Effectiveness:** The individual assesses the potential as to whether or not adopting appropriate IPC practice will serve to enhance their level of protection against contracting an infection measured against failing to adopt such.
- **Self-Efficacy:** Within the context of IPC the individual draws upon their past experience and knowledge as a measure of and the level of risk they would place themselves with regards to acquiring an infection in the future.
- **Fear:** Where the undertaking of IPC practice is concerned, the individual will try to balance the psychological and emotional effects between their id and the superego measured against adopting appropriate practice or not as a result of ego mediation.

1.8 EGOCENTRISM

Egocentric behaviour (Ogden 2019; Bocian et al. 2020) may be described as a self-centred, self-fulfilling and self-orientated behaviour without consideration of others, leading to an overrated self-perception of their position or role. For example, beliefs around role, status and the undertaking of tasks deemed as being below one's station is an interesting case in point in health care, with some groups believing that other groups should tidy up after a procedure. List 1.2 offers some examples of egocentric behaviours.

LIST 1.2 EXAMPLES OF EGOCENTRISM AND IPC

- **Example 1:** Rationalised beliefs that their IPC practice is always safe and superior to others.
- **Example 2:** Hypocrisy where the individual fails to perceive blatant irregularities between what they profess to be correct and use their authority to override the suggestions of others who may in reality offer more appropriate perspectives related to the application of IPC practices.
- **Example 3:** Where the individual chooses not to recognise the importance of adopting appropriate standard precautions because they believe they know better within the context of the right place, the time, in the right way and applied to the right person.
- **Example 4:** The sanctimonious individual who believes they are professionally, ethically and morally superior to colleagues irrespective of who those colleagues are and as such where IPC practices are concerned, where they believe they are right despite any evidence that would indicate otherwise.

1.9 ARROGANCE

Arrogance may be perceived as an attribute within an individual's personality equating to perceptions of superiority (Cleary et al. 2015) that may also be consistent with type A personality. Certainly, Berger (2002) and Milyavsky et al. (2017) indicate that arrogance can be problematic. Within this context, List 1.3 offers examples that may impact upon IPC practice.

LIST 1.3 EXAMPLES OF ARROGANCE THAT MAY IMPACT UPON SAFE IPC PRACTICE

- I practice IPC my way irrespective of what you think!
- Who are you to challenge me over my IPC practice!
- A rationalised belief in their superiority where their IPC practice is concerned!
- A rationalised belief that their appointment makes them more knowledgeable where their IPC practice is concerned!
- A rationalised belief that they are right even when they are wrong!

1.10 MICROAGGRESSIONS

Williams (2019) sets out a number of key assertions related to microaggressions as presented in List 1.4.

LIST 1.4 MICROAGGRESSION ASSERTIONS

- Microaggressions are interpreted negatively by most or all minority group members
- Microaggressions reflect implicitly prejudicial and implicitly aggressive motives
- Microaggressions can be validly assessed using only respondents' subjective reports
- Microaggressions exert an adverse impact on recipients' mental health

Cited directly from Williams (2019)

Microaggressions can be experienced by any group of individuals, including race, religion gender, sexuality orientation, disability, age, class or profession. In further defining micro-aggression, they can be identified in three main categories (List 1.5).

LIST 1.5 MAIN CATEGORIES OF MICROAGGRESSIONS: VERBAL AND NON-VERBAL

- Microassaults: Which in general are deliberate with the intention of threatening, intimidating, to exclude, to insult or to humiliate.
- Microinsults: Which are reflective of stereotypes, insensitivity, rudeness, to disrespect, to make assumptions or demeaning.
- Microinvalidations: Which can be exclusionary, put down in nature, oppressive, stigmatisation, to deny a voice, to discredit or to show disinterest.

Health Essentials (2022).

List 1.6 identifies ways in which these could be applied to IPC.

LIST 1.6 EXAMPLE MICROAGGRESSIONS LINKED TO IPC

- *"As you are a new student nurse and have only just started your course, I guess you will not know much about IPC!"*
  This microaggression is the assumption that because the student has just started their course that they will lack knowledge of IPC. This does not consider previous experience and knowledge of IPC.
- *"As they are senior to you, they have more knowledge and experience than you regarding IPC."*
  The microaggression here is the linking of seniority to knowledge and experience. Just because an individual is more senior, it does not follow that they will be more knowledgeable and experienced. This microaggression may be demeaning and oppressive.

Microaggression can have negative consequences and the individuals affected may feel like it's a "death by a thousand cuts" (Alva and Montoya 2021) (List 1.7).

LIST 1.7 THE BIOPSYCHOSOCIAL CONSEQUENCES OF MICROAGGRESSIONS

Physical	Psychological	Social
Feeling exhausted	Reduced communications	Self-isolation
Failure to thrive	Increased stress	Raised sickness rates
Reduces self-care	Changes in behaviour	Marginalisation
Increased risk of errors	Poorly thought out language	Cultural isolation
Physical illness	Stereotyping others	Religious intolerance
Sleep deprivation	Inner conflicts	Breaches of human rights:
Suicide	Irritability	Articles 1, 3, 5, 9, 14
Eating habit changes	Paranoia	Colour blindness

In consideration of the previous section, reflect upon the following:

1. Think of an occasion when you were subjected to a microaggression.
   How did it make you feel?
   In retrospect, what response did you make or should you have made at the time in reflecting back?
2. Think of a time when you made a microaggression towards another person.
   Were you aware of such at the time?
   How did the other person react?
   How did you feel at the time, and how do you feel about what you did now?
3. In what ways will you in the future be more aware of microaggressions?
   What behavioural changes will you make to ensure that you do not inflict microaggressions on others in the future?

Finally, it is interesting to note that within the health and social care, microaggressions may be more common than is generally realised and can take many forms (Farris et al. 2017; Spencer 2017; Overland et al. 2019; Molina et al. 2020; Ackerman-Barger et al. 2021).

1.11 DECISION-MAKING

Decision-making can be defined as the reaching of a conclusion either individually or through a group consensus regarding any potential set of behavioural actions (Schoemaker and Russo 2016).

However, this definition does not reflect how such a process evolves so as to ensure that transmission of infection is reduced through the behaviours of those involved in the provision of health and social care. Elliott et al. (2016) and Standing (2017) both identify adaptations of the cognitive continuum as being useful in serving to facilitate levels of decision-making which can, if applied appropriately, lead to more valid and reliable decision-making.

Diagram 1.3 reflects an adaptation of Hamm's (1984) work as set out in Dowie and Elstein (1996).

LIST 1.8 DIALOGUE TO DIAGRAM 1.3

Level 6: Intuitive informed decision-making is essentially subjective and thus will lack both validity and reliability. As such, it is a highly questionable decision-making strategy in isolation because, as Hogarth (2010) identifies, "the essence of intuition or intuitive responses is that they are reached with little apparent effort, and typically without conscious awareness. They involve little or no conscious deliberation."

Level 5: Peer informed decision-making can constitute subjectivity in the transference of information in that an individual is likely to pass on what they believe

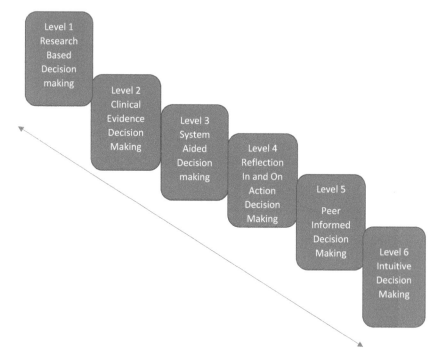

DIAGRAM 1.3   The Cognitive Continuum, a Decision-Making Process

you should know, which may not actually be what you need to know. However, there is evidence to suggest that handovers are "inaccurate, incomplete, and biased may lead to many errors, mislead nursing practices, and increase patient complications" (Sarvestani et al. 2015).

Level 4: Reflection informed decision-making, whether it be in or on action can constitute a useful resource for future practice if it is undertaken appropriately, where individuals must be open to both their positive practice and to aspects of their practice which require development. However, it must also be recognised that reflection is a subjective and ambiguous process (Clara 2015) and, as such, must always be perceived within that context when used in decision-making.

Level 3: System-aided informed decision-making can constitute an objective perspective where the provision of information is concerned if such systems are appropriately maintained, serviced and calibrated. However, where systems are concerned, it must always be borne in mind that if they can go wrong, then there will always be the potential for such to occur, and as such, regular maintenance and management is vital (Bahreini et al. 2018). Therefore, the objectivity of medical systems will only be maintained if such occurs.

Level 2: Clinical decision-making must always be objective in nature if it is to be valid and reliable and facilitate safe practice. Within an IPC context, when an infection is suspected, objective clinical decision-making would be the taking of an individual's vital signs, which would include temperature, pule rate, respirations rate, blood pressure, blood sugar, urinalysis, dehydration, confusion, agitation, productive cough, amongst other signs and symptoms.

Level 1: Research informed decision-making has the potential to constitute objective evidence so long as the work has, for example, been peer reviewed, a valid research process is followed and is ethical. However, even if these are apparent, it will not necessarily guarantee the validity and reliability of published materials as Ioannidis (2005), Fenelli (2009), Nurunnabi and Hossian (2018), Kang and Hwang (2020) all identify, which is not only concerning but brings in to question the appropriateness of decision-making using published materials, whether they be quantitative, qualitative methodologies in nature, or which statistical approaches are used, inferential or descriptive. In essence, where effective decision-making is concerned, none of the levels within Diagram 1.3 should be used in isolation. Rather, a combination of such will enhance the potential towards providing a valid and reliable IPC decision-making process, which is why Hamm referred to his model as a continuum.

1.12 WILL NOT HAPPEN TO ME

The principle of individuals believing "it will not happen to me" irrespective of whatever form of IPC practice they may undertake constitutes a defence mechanism which will serve to protect the individual (Perrotta 2020). This acts to reduce psychological conflict, stress or emotionally harmful experiences (Walker and McCabe 2020), which would allow the individual to carry out behaviours which may or may not constitute safe practice. Such a belief is a rationalized and cognitively economic process as it most certainly may well happen to them where their IPC practice is not up to standard.

1.13 LOCUS OF CONTROL

Locus of control (Barley 2016) consists of two dimensions:

Internal: Where a partnership exists between the individual and the practitioner. Such partnerships reflect the equality of all parties involved and reflective of a biopsychosocial perspective.

External: This is where the individual is expected to be unquestioning, compliant and submissive to the demands of practitioners. Such an approach being reflective of a biomedical perspective.

However, within the context of IPC practice, this should reflect the context and an internal locus of control where the individual should feel free and able to question and offer their thoughts with regards to ensuring that safe and appropriate IPC practice is undertaken without fear of ridicule, retribution or falling standards of care.

1.14 COMPENSATORY RISK-TAKING BEHAVIOUR

In health and social care, professionals are consistently presented with competing requirements and demands related to their practice (Carayon and Durses 2008; Yunus and Mahajr 2015). In such situations, practitioners are confronted on a regular basis with having to make decisions based upon the quality of their practice measured against a number of factors (List 1.8). Generally, factors such as shortages of staff and/or equipment, delays in decision-making, excessive workloads, long working hours, concerns about safety can make working in health care an arduous undertaking. There is a need to draw a balance between meeting an individual's needs measured against adopting safe IPC practice. Lists 1.9 and 1.10 present example factors and considerations relevant to this concept.

LIST 1.9 EXAMPLES OF FACTORS PRACTITIONERS MUST TAKE INTO ACCOUNT RELATED TO COMPENSATORY RISK-TAKING

- The individual's specific healthcare need(s).
- The severity of the individual's healthcare problem(s).
- The degree to which an individual can care for themselves.
- The level of input required from the practitioner.
- The total number of individuals the practitioner has been allocated to care for.
- Having to measure one individual's need against others' needs.
- The amount of time a given individual will need to spend with the individual in respect of their care needs.

LIST 1.10 REFLECTIVE FACTORS THAT PRACTITIONERS MUST CONSIDER WITH REGARDS TO COMPENSATORY RISK-TAKING

- Who are the individuals to whom I have been allocated?
- What are the individuals physical, psychological and social needs?
- When will the practitioner need to undertake the specific interventions required?
- Where within the practitioner's sphere of working is the individual located?
- How will it be ensured that the appropriate resources required for the care of a given individual are available?
- Why all of the above are important?

- Who Says So being the most important component of all of the stages within this reflective approach because each of the above stages must be supported with appropriate evidence.

(Extracts from Elliott in Jasper et al. 2013)

1.15 BULLYING AND HARASSMENT

Bullying and harassment in the workplace (Shiwani and Elenin 2010; Szutenbach 2013; Akella 2016; De Sio et al. 2020) occur in most workplaces, including healthcare organisations (Karatza et al. 2016; Wallace and Gipson 2017). It can have a significant impact upon an individual's mental and physical health and wellbeing (Wolke and Lereya 2015) and can also impact upon the safety of those who seek their interventions (Lever et al. 2019). Bullying and harassment can have an impact upon an individual's psychosocial health and wellbeing (Asrar et al. 2021). Addressing bullying and harassment is an ongoing challenge for organisations and is influenced by a complex interplay of organisational culture and leadership and the associated factors around these. The drivers of bullying and the factors that motivate an individual to bully and harass others are complex and can lead to low morale, reduced self-esteem and anxiety, resulting in loss of motivation related to their IPC practice.

In concluding this chapter, I have attempted to present a number of psychosocial theories and approaches that can have an influence upon not only the perception of IPC but also implication for the resulting practices.

1.16 REFERENCES

Ackerman-Barger, K., Jacobs, N., Orozco, R. and London, M. (2021), Addressing microaggressions in academic health: A workshop for inclusive excellence, *Journal of the Association of American Medical Colleges*, Available Online at: www.ncbi.nlm.nih.gov/pmc/articles/PMC7880252/pdf/mep_2374-8265.11103.pdf Accessed: 10 July 2022.

Akella, D. (2016), Workplace bullying: Not a manager's right? *Journal of Workplace Rights*, 6 (1), 1–10.

Alva, A. and Montoya, E. (2021), Posted by morningsignout, *The Effects of Microaggressions on One's Health, Medicine and Pharmacy*, Available Online at: https://sites.uci.edu/morning-signout/2021/03/09/the-effects-of-microaggressions-on-ones-health/ Accessed: 10 July 2022.

Asrar, H., Amen, U., Sumayya, U. and Butt, A. (2021), Impact of workforce bullying on psychological wellbeing of doctors in health care sector of Pakistan, *Journal of Entrepreneurship, Management and Innovation*, 3 (2), 429–450.

Ayers, S. and De Visser, R. (2018), *Psychology for Medicine and Healthcare* (2nd ed.), London, SAGE Publications, 226–227.

Bahreini, R., Doshmangir, L. and Imani, A. (2018), Factors affecting medical equipment maintenance management: A systematic review, *Journal of Clinical and Diagnostic Research*, 12 (4), IC01–IC07.

Barley, E. (2016), *Health Psychology in Nursing Practice*, London, SAGE Publications, 105.

Barnhart, J. (1972), Freud's pleasure principle and the death urge, *The Southwestern Journal of Philosophy*, 3 (1), 113–120.

Berger, A. (2002), Arrogance among physicians, *Academic Medicine*, 77 (2), 145–147.

Bocian, K., Baryla, W. and Wojciszke, B. (2020), Egocentrism shapes moral judgements, *Social and Personality Psychology Compass*, 14 (912), 1–14.

Chandu, V., Ligameneni, K., Pachava, S., Baddam, V. and Marella, Y. (2022), The influence of dissonance and assessment reactivity in improving adherence to COVID-19 precautionary measures: A cluster randomized controlled trial, *International Dental Journal*, 72 (2), 141–148.

Clarà, M. (2015), What is reflection? Looking for clarity in an ambiguous notion, *Journal of Teacher Education*, 66 (3), 261–271.

Cleary, M., Walter, G., Sayers, J., Lopez, V. and Hungerford, C. (2015), Arrogance in the workplace: Implications for mental health nurses, *Issues in Mental Health Nursing*, 36, 266–271.

Crayon, P. and Durses, A. (2008), Nursing workload and patient safety: A human factors engineering perspective, in Hugues, R. (ed.), *Patient Safety and Quality: An Evidenced- Based handbook for Nurses*, Available Online at: www.ncbi.nlm.nih.gov/books/NBK2657/pdf/Bookshelf_NBK2657.pdf Accessed: 28 July 2022.

Creedon, S. (2006), Infection control: Behavioural issues for healthcare workers, *Clinical Governance: An International Journal*, 11 (4), 316–325.

De Sio, S., Cedrone, F. and Buomprisco, G. (2020), Bullying at work and work-related stress in healthcare workers: A cross sectional study, *Annali di igiene: Medicina Preventiva e di Comunità*, 32 (2), 109–116.

Elliott, P. (2009), *Infection Control: A Psychosocial Approach to Changing Practice*, Boca Raton, Taylor and Francis, 5–9, 12–13, 73–99.

Elliott, P. (2013), Moving from clinical supervision to person-centred development: A paradigm change, in Jasper, M., Rosser, M. and Mooney, G. (eds.), Professional *Development, Reflection and Decision-Making in Nursing and Health Care*, Chichester, Wiley Blackwell, 168–203.

Elliott, P., Storr, J. and Jeanes, A. (2016), *In Infection Prevention and Control: Perceptions and Perspectives*, Boca Raton, Taylor and Francis, 63–77.

Farris, T., Lee, Y.-M. and Hartman, E. (2017), Racial microaggressions within the field of nursing, Available Online at: https://core.ac.uk/download/pdf/232976992.pdf Accessed: 28 July 2022.

Fenelli, D. (2009), How many scientists fabricate and Falsify research? A systematic review and meta-analysis of survey data, *PLoS One*, 4 (5), e5738.

Festinger, L. (1962), Cognitive dissonance, *Scientific American*, 207, 93–102.

Freud, S. (1981), New introductory lectures on paychoanalysis, in Slack, J. (ed.), *Introduction to Psychology, Psychology of the Person (Unit 2): Psychodynamics*, Milton Keynes, Open University.

Gammon, J. and Hunt, J. (2020), COVID-19 and hand hygiene: The vital importance of hand drying, *British Journal of Nursing*, 29 (17), 1003–1006.

Hamm, R. M. (1984), Clinical intuition and clinical analysis: Expertise and the cognitive continuum, in Dowie, J. and Elstein, A. (1996 eds.), *Professional Judgement: A Reader in Clinical Decision Making*, Cambridge, Cambridge University Press, 78–105.

Health Essentials (2022), What are microaggressions, Available Online at: https://health.clevelandclinic.org/what-are-microaggressions-and-examples/ Accessed: 28 July 2022.

Hogarth, R. (2010), Intuition: A challenge for psychological research on decision making, *Psychological Inquiry*, 21 (4), 338–353.

Ioannidis, J. (2005), Why most published research findings are false, *PLoS Medicine*, 2 (8), 0696–0701.

Jefferson, A., Bortolotti, L. and Kuzmanovic, B. (2017), What is unrealistic optimism? *Consciousness and Cognition*, 50, 3–11.

Kang, E. and Hwang, H-J. (2020), The consequences of data fabrication and falsification among researchers, *Journal of Research and Publication Ethics*, 1 (2), 7–10.

Karabatos, I., Tsagkaris, C. and Kalachanis, K. (2021), All roads lead to Rome: Aspects of public health in ancient Rome, *Le Infezioni Medicina*, 3, 488–491.

Karatza, C., Zyga., Tziaferi, S. and Prezerakos, P. (2016), Workplace bullying and general health status among the nursing staff of a Greek public hospitals, *Annals of General Psychiatry*, 15 (7), 1–7.

Lever, I., Dyball, D., Greenberg, N. and Stevelink, S. (2019), Health consequences of bullying in the health workplace: A systematic review, *Journal of Advanced Nursing*, 75, 3195–3209.

McLeod, S. (2016), *Id, Ego and Superego* (updated from 2007), Retrieved form Simple Psychology, Available Online at: https://cpb-ca-c1.wpmucdn.com/myriverside.sd43.bc.ca/dist/b/55/files/2017/10/simplypsychology.org-psyche-10czxts.pdf Accessed: 28 July 2022.

Milyavsky, M., Kruglanski, A., Chernikova, M. and Schori-Eyal, N. (2017), Evidence for arrogance: On the relative importance of expertise, outcome and manner, *PLoS One*, 12 (7), 1–31.

Molina, M., Landry, A., Chary, A. and Burnett-Bowie, S.-A. (2020), *Addressing the Elephant in the Room: Microaggression in Medicine, American College of Emergency Physicians*, Annals of Emergency Medicine, Available Online at: https://medicine.umich.edu/sites/default/files/downloads/microaggressions_0.pdf Accessed: 28 July 2022.

Nurunnabi, M. and Hossain, M. (2018), Data falsification and question on academic integrity, *Accountability in Research*, 26 (2), 108–122.

Ogden, J. (2019), *Health Psychology* (6th ed.), London, McGraw Hill, 4–10 and 31.

Overland, M., Zumsteg, J., Lindo, E., Sholas, M., Montenegro, R., Campelia, G. and Feature Editor: Mukherjee, D. (2019), Microaggressions in clinical training and practice, *American Academy of Physical Medicine*, 11, 1004–1012.

Parker, J. and Davies, B. (2020), No blame no gain? From a no blame culture to a responsibility culture in medicine, *Journal of Applied Philosophy*, 37 (4), 646–660.

Perrotta, G. (2020), Human mechanisms of psychological defence: Definitions, historical and psychodynamic contexts, classifications and clinical profiles, *International Journal of Neurorehabilitation*, 7 (360), 1–7.

Roth, I. and Firsby, J. (1992), *Perception and Representation: A Cognitive Approach*, Buckingham, Open University Press, 18–23.

Sabet Sarvestani, R., Moattari, M., Nasrabadi, A., Momennasab, M. and Yektatalab, S. (2015), Challenges of nursing handover: A qualitative study, *Clinical Nursing Research*, 24 (3), 234–252.

Schoemaker, P. and Russo, J. (2016), Decision-making, in Augier, M. and Teece, D. (eds.), *The Palgrave Encyclopedia of Strategic Management*, London, Palgrave Macmillan.

Shiwani, M. and Elenin, H. (2010), Bullying and harassment at workplace: Are we aware? *Journal of Pakistan Medical Association*, 60 (7), 516–517.

Siegfried, W. (2014), The formation and structure of the human psyche, *Athene Noctua: Undergraduate Philosophy Journal*, Available Online at: www.fau.edu/athenenoctua/pdfs/William%20Siegfried.pdf Accessed: 30 March 2022.

Smith, P., Watkins, K. and Hewlett, A. (2012), Infection control through the ages, *American Journal of Infection Control*, 40, 35–42.

Spencer, M, (2017), Microaggressions and social work practice: Education, and research, *Journal of Ethnic and Cultural Diversity in Social Work*, 26, 1–2, 1–5.

Standing, M. (2017), *Clinical Judgement and Decision Making in Nursing* (3rd ed.), London, SAGE Publications, 6–8.

Szutenbach, M. (2013), Bullying in nursing, *Journal of Christian Nursing*, 30 (1), 17–23.

Turabian, J. (2018), Patient-centered care and biopsychosocial model, *Trends in General Practice*, 1 (3), 1–2.

Walker, G. and McCabe, T. (2020), Psychological defence mechanisms during the COVID-19 pandemic: A case series, *The European Journal of Psychiatry*, 35 (1), 41–45.

Wallace, S. and Gipson, K. (2017), Bullying in healthcare: A disruptive force linked to compromised patient safety, *Pennsylvania Patient Safety Advisory*, 14 (2), 64–70.

Weinstein, N. (1982), Unrealistic optimism about susceptibility to health problems, *Journal of Behavioural Medicine*, 5, 441–460.

Welkenhuysen, M., Evers-Kiebooms, G., Decruyenaere, M. and Vanden Berghe, H. (1996), Unrealistic optimism and genetic risk, *Psychology and Health*, 11, 479–492.

Williams, L. (2012), Starting out—discovering the psychology behind good infection control, *Nursing Standard*, 26 (26), 29.

Williams, M. (2019), Microaggressions: Clarification, evidence, and impact, *Perspectives on Psychological Science*, 15 (1), 3–26.

Wolke, D. and Lereya, S. (2015), Long-term effects of bullying, *British Medical Journal*, 100, 879–885.

Yunus, J. and Mahajar, A. (2015), Work overload, role ambiguity and role boundary and its effect on burnout among nurses of public hospitals in Malaysia, *International Journal of Research in Humanities and Social Studies*, 2 (10), 18–25.

The Psychosocial Nature of Infection Prevention and Control

2

Paul Elliott

Contents

2.1 INTRODUCTION

This chapter is in two parts and is concerned with a deeper exploration of the psychosocial factors relevant to IPC with the term psychosocial first coming to prominence in the 1890s (Hayward 2012). Part 1 outlines several factors related to the psychosocial nature of IPC. It includes a consideration of rights-based approaches, including the relevance of the human rights act to IPC. Part 2 outlines a number of strategies that may facilitate future IPC practice and the transmission and subsequent acquisition of infection.

2.1.1 Part 1

To begin, with regards to processes that may impact negatively upon individuals' safe and appropriate IPC practice, I will focus on the psychosocial factors that may indirectly reduce a practitioner's approach to safety. List 2.1 sets out a number of these psychosocially related factors concerning the perceptions of health workers.

DOI: 10.1201/9781003379393-3

LIST 2.1 PSYCHOSOCIAL FACTORS THAT CAN SERVE TO INDIRECTLY FACILITATE UNSAFE IPC PRACTICE

- Staff feeling that their personal safety is at risk.
- Staff feeling colleagues and management care little about them so long as the workload is completed.
- Staff feeling they have no voice and are unable to express their thoughts and feelings due to managerial and employer reactions and responses.
- Staff feeling their efforts go unrecognised and are unappreciated through receiving only negative responses or receiving dismissive behaviour.
- Staff feeling demotivated through the employer and managers' failure to recognise their needs. For example, the failing to ensure that staff take their breaks and thus being unable to maintain their nutritional and fluid balance.
- Staff feeling that they are not being treated with respect, fairness, understanding or empathy.
- Staff feeling that they are treated equally in respect of racism, sexism, ageism and freedom from religious/cultural disparity.
- Staff feeling that they are treated in a humanistic way and feel fulfilled with regards to being perceived as a person as opposed to being subjected to stereotyping and dehumanisation.
- Staff feeling that they will not be placed in situations where their health and wellbeing may be at risk without the provision of appropriate support and guidance from a biopsychosocial perspective.

It is within this context that matters of human rights enter into the fray. If individuals believe they are not being treated fairly, they may perceive that their human rights are being violated. List 2.2 sets out elements of the Human Rights Act that could be considered of relevance to IPC.

LIST 2.2 ELEMENTS OF THE HUMAN RIGHTS ACT RELATED TO IPC (United Nations 1948)

- **Obligations to secure rights and freedoms:** Every individual has the right to expect such to be maintained with regards to the maintenance of IPC practices.
- **Right to life:** Every individual has the right to have not only their life protected but also their future quality of life where the safe application of IPC standards are concerned.
- **Prohibition of torture:** Individuals have a right to be protected from physical, psychological and social harm, pain and suffering through the appropriate implementation of IPC procedures.
- **Freedom of expression:** Every individual has the right to question or challenge others irrespective of who they are where either their own or others' health, safety and welfare is concerned with regards to their standards of IPC practice.

- **Prohibition of discrimination:** Every individual has the right not to be exposed to discrimination with regards to the application of IPC on an equal basis.

Considering the requirement to meet individuals' human rights in the context of standard precautions yields some interesting considerations; several of which are presented in List 2.3. The reader may have others to add to this list.

LIST 2.3 STANDARD PRECAUTIONS AND HUMAN RIGHTS

- Recognising the need to adopt standard precautions and the implications of failure to do so and its contribution to unsafe practice that if recognised must be responded to (Blair 2021) through a professional intervention so that the individual recognises the need to adopt appropriate standard precautions.
- Adherence with hand hygiene evidence base (Bimback 2017).
- Access to disposable aprons and gloves for single use only (Wigglesworth 2019).
- Clothing and uniforms and the potential risk of both the acquisition and transmission of microbes (Aljohani et al. 2017; Owen et al. 2021) within all environments.
- Sharps must be handled safely due to their potential to cause harm (Dulon et al. 2020; Hussein and Saad 2021).
- Spillages must be dealt with appropriately due to their potential to cause harm or have toxic effects. For example, where blood and body fluids are concerned (Grimmond et al. 2020).
- The importance of personal hygiene for appropriate professionally orientated social interactions (Ali et al. 2018).

Failures related to any of the previously cited considerations may lead to a perceived breach of any or all the articles in List 2.2 and from a psychosocial perspective may precipitate feelings of stress, anxiety and distress in an individual. Further, standard precautions could be considered to constitute a universal set of prescriptive rules that can impact either positively or negatively upon an individual's health or social care intervention(s) and future quality of life. However, there is evidence to indicate that prescriptive rules are not always adhered to as articulated (Reason et al. 1998; Lawton and Parker 2002; Carthey et al. 2011; Medical Legal Concepts LLC 2016). Considering some of the psychosocial theories and approaches outlined in Chapter 1 concerning personality, here it could be stated that the id remains infantile in its functioning (McLeod 2016), and individuals tend to dislike being told what to do (Bouchoucha and Moore 2017) unless the individual perceives there is something to be gained either in terms of gratification or pleasure. If we go further and link this gratification or pleasure-seeking principle to that of Freud's ideas (Mutiah 2010), it may go some way to offering an explanation, from a psychosocial perspective, why individuals do not always adhere to prescriptive rules in that, for example, an individual may perceive completing their workload within a given time span as constituting a pleasurable experience and thus cognitively put aside their need to adopt standard precautions within the context of such being a set of prescriptive rules. Further, it is also inevitable, in failing to adhere to standard precautions as prescriptive rules, the processes of cognitive dissonance (Festinger 1962), unrealistic optimism (Weinstein 1982) and cognitive economy (Roth and Frisby 1992) will also be impacting upon the individual's non-adherent behaviour. Considering non-adherence with guidelines through a purely psychosocial lens does throw up some interesting areas that are worth considering by those developing and implementing guidance. However, as Carthey et al. (2011) highlight, the reasons for noncompliance are multifactorial. The chapters in this book that focus on human factors probe even further into the reasons behind noncompliance and explore how human factors approaches that draw on the psychosocial can help to overcome these challenges.

2.1.2 Part 2

Part 1 offers several approaches that may serve to facilitate individuals' undertaking of safe and appropriate IPC practice. In Part 2, the focus is on reflection. Reflection is a process that can be undertaken with regards to an individual's IPC practice both in and on action (Jasper 2003; Wain 2017). It is important to recognise that reflection is a process which is intended to facilitate individuals to be able to recognise within an environment that they feel safe, how they can psychosocially enhance their awareness with regards to any aspect of their beliefs, attitudes or behaviour. List 2.4 offers an example of a reflective process linked to IPC.

LIST 2.4 A REFLECTIVE PROCESS

Who: Who can support me in reducing the risk of IPC errors and misjudgments?

What: What evidence can I identify that will serve to reduce my potential for errors or misjudgments with regards to IPC?

When: When am I most at risk of IPC errors or misjudgments—what can I do to offset the potential for such risks?

Where: Where does my working environment contribute to my potential towards IPC errors or misjudgments, and how can I work towards ensuring that my environment has less impact upon my potential for IPC errors and misjudgments?

How: What actions can I take towards ensuring my potential for making IPC errors and misjudgments is reduced as far as is possible?

Why: Why in the past have I allowed things to affect my perception of what does or does not constitute safe IPC practice?

However, the final step in this process is the most important element:

Who Says So: How will I know that my subjective reflections are valid and reliable? What objective evidence can I obtain to validate and demonstrate the reliability of my reflections? If the "who says so" element of this reflective process is not undertaken, then it is likely that one's reflection will be perceived as subjective conjecture.

(Adapted from Elliott in Jasper et al. 2013)

A further model of reflection is an adaptation (List 2.5) of Goodman's (1984) levels of reflection as set out in Jasper (2003). The value of Goodman's model is that it sets out specific levels which can serve to give the individual some direction as to what they might wish to give thought to regarding their reflections.

LIST 2.5 AN ADAPTATION OF GOODMAN'S MODEL OF REFLECTION RELATED TO IPC

Level 1 Reflection:
Within this context, your reflective focus should be able to demonstrate a sound factual knowledge and descriptive understanding of your skills related to IPC supported by appropriate academic evidence in order to support your reflections.

Level 2 Reflection:
Within this level of reflection, you would be expected to be able to clearly demonstrate achievement of level 1. Further, at this level, your reflective focus should centre on having an understanding of the implications and consequences of your IPC practice and be able to evaluate your problem-solving and decision-making process in relation to such. Further, you should be able to display an ability to understand the concepts related to your attitudes, beliefs and stereotypes that might impact upon your ability to undertake safe IPC practice as well as being able to demonstrate an understanding of the biopsychosocal model and its implications for your individualised IPC practice and offer published evidence to support this.

Level 3 Reflection:
Within this level of reflection, you would be expected to be able to demonstrate achievement of both levels 1 and 2. Further, at this level you should be able to recognise and evaluate the conceptual nature of your knowledge, skills and IPC practice. At this level of reflection, you would be expected to question and challenge current thinking, the status quo, current clinical practice and the theory that is alledged to underpin such and to offer alternatives supported by published evidence.

(Adapted from Goodman 1984 in Jasper 2003)

1. **Questioning, challenging, raising concerns and speaking up** is something that all health and social care professionals must do in relation to observing suboptimal practice irrespective of the profession or appointment and no matter how senior or junior the individual is whose compliance is of concern (Okuyama et al. 2014; Ion et al. 2016; Wong and Ginsburg 2017). However, if practitioners fail to allow and involve individuals to do this, they could be perceived as being in contravention of peoples' human rights as set out in List 2.2. No health or social care professional should ever ethically consider themselves above being questioned or challenged by colleagues, others or participating in their own care (Vahdat et al. 2014; Smith and Mee 2017; Rodrigo-Rincon et al. 2022). Such questioning and challenging of practitioners' IPC practice must always be accepted in a professional manner.

2. **Whistle-blowing** can be another way of facilitating appropriate IPC practice and is an appropriate behaviour regarding inappropriate, unsafe or unethical behaviour occuring in the workplace (Chen 2019; Armitage and Nellums 2020). Undertaking such a process can serve to facilitate safe IPC practice as it serves to identify those practitioners whose standards of professional practice are or have fallen below what is considered acceptable and as such will put others at risk. Certainly, this can be related to a breach of article 2 of the Human Rights Act (List 2.2) because any drop in standards precipitates harm to others and must be brought to the attention of the relevant authority. Failure to blow the whistle serves to make the individual as culpable as the practitioner who practices below an acceptable standard, albeit the ability to blow the whistle will be influenced by many factors, including an organisation's culture.

3. **Allocated time** for professional development within practitioners' working hours should be an essential responsibility of all employers and not simply left to practitioners having to undertake within their own time. Allocated time is of benefit to employers to ensure practitioners maintain their professional registration to enhance their knowledge and skills. During working hours, many barriers exist, but a more supportive approach on the part of employers could have beneficial outcomes (Mlambo et al. 2021). This may also provide a forum in which to provide more continuing professional development opportunities.

4. **Staying away from work when unwell** will reduce the risk of both the acquisition and transmission of infection. Individuals may feel the need to "struggle in" to work despite feeling unwell and potentially infectious (Collins and Cartwright 2012; Mekonnen et al. 2018) whilst offering dissonance-based rationalisations for doing so. Such behaviour, often referred to as presenteeism, can be in contravention of their professional code of conduct, health and safety law and demonstrates a disregard for the health and wellbeing of others. Managing individuals who attend work whilst unwell is a challenge, yet being subject to some level of managerial intervention which may not be of a disciplinary recourse but rather of an empathetic and supportive nature is important. Policy reiteration and reinforcement could be used in a humanistic manner by explaining to the individual that they need to go home with a copy of the relevant policy and asked not to return until they are well again. However, within the context of protecting the individual, from a psychosocial perspective, Taylor et al. (2021) highlights the potential for those who are present at work whilst sick to be subjected to mistreatment because of their constituting a risk to colleagues. As such, although the individual has attended work inappropriately, there exists a duty of care to them in the form of protecting them from adverse and unprofessional psychosocial abuse in respect of bullying, stereotyping, harassment or violence (Baguena et al. 2011; Meyer and Kirsten 2014; Elliott et al. 2016; Bulut and Hihi 2021). The COVID-19 pandemic revealed many examples of the complexities of presenteeism and the personal, organizational and occupational factors that influence people's decisions about whether they should attend work or stay away (Kinman 2019).

5. **Pricking the moral conscience** may, from a psychosocial perspective, constitute a means of facilitating, along with other strategies, improved adherence to

IPC practice. Within the context of conscience, Birchley (2011) offers an interesting discussion regarding the conscience related to having the right to object where the right to defy authority is concerned. However, in contrast, Cleary and Lees (2019) suggest what can be perceived as a different perspective on conscience where it relates to acting morally and ethically as the guardians of such where the provision of care is concerned, which can be perceived as including the appropriate undertaking of standard precautions (List 2.3). Despite these differing perspectives, pricking a colleague's conscience in a professional and humanistic manner may have beneficial outcomes.

6. **Leading by example** may serve to facilitate the IPC practice and particularly where the leader is respected and perceived by others as caring and humanistic in the manner of their leadership (Oliver 2006; West et al. 2015; Maxwell 2017). Certainly, a team observing a valued and humanistic leader are more likely to be predisposed to following their example than someone they perceive to be an autocratic boss, as is exemplified by Chudasama (2021) and who clearly identifies that a leadership style will serve to facilitate the best in individuals.

Those working in the field of IPC undertake a journey on their route to becoming a competent IPC professional. Many national bodies outline such competencies to support this journey. The World Health Organization (WHO 2020) in their description of IPC core competencies refer to the knowledge, skills and attitudes required for an IPC professional to practice with an in-depth understanding of situations, using reasoning, critical thinking, reflection and analysis to inform assessment and decision-making in the prevention and control of healthcare-associated infection and antimicrobial resistance. In concluding this chapter, it has been my intention to stimulate thinking and discussion in relation to the psychosocial issues related to IPC, including the importance of reflection. It is my hope that this has generated thinking related to your own attitudes, beliefs, and practice as you move forward in your own journey as a professional.

2.2 REFERENCES

Ali, G., Mohamed, N. and Mahdy, A. (2018), Personal hygiene and taking into account the preventative measures and safety among healthcare providers, *International Journal of Advanced Nursing Studies*, 7 (1), 44–54.

Aljohani, Y., Alumtadares, M., Alfaifi, K., Madhoun, M., Albahiti, M. and Al-Hazmi, N. (2017), Uniform-related infection control practices of dental students, *Infection and Drug Resistance*, 10, 135–142.

Armitage, R. and Nellums, L. (2020), Whistleblowing and patient safety during COVID-19, *The Lancet*, 24, Available Online at: https://doi.org/10.1016/j.eclinm.2020.100425 Accessed: 6 December 2022.

Baguena, M., Belena, M., Toldos, M. and Martinez, D. (2011), Psychological harassment in the workplace: Methods of evaluation and prevalence, *The Open Criminology Journal*, 4, 102–108.

Bimback, D. (2017), The importance of hand washing, *Infectious Diseases, The Lancet*, 17 (8), 811.

Birchley, G. (2011), A case for conscience in healthcare practice, *Journal of Medical Ethics*, 38 (1), 13–17.

Blair, W., Kable, A., Palazzi, K., Courtney-Pratt, H., Doran, E. and Oldmeadow, C. (2021), Nurses' perspectives of recognising and responding to unsafe practice by their peers: A national cross-sectional survey, *Journal of Clinical Nursing*, 30, 1168–1183.

Bouchoucha, S. and Moore, K. (2017), Standard precautions but no standard adherence, *Australian Nursing and Midwifery Journal*, 24 (8), 38.

Bulut, S. and Hihi, S. (2021), Bullying in the workplace: The psychological causes and effects of bullying in the workplace, *Clinical Research in Psychology*, 4 (1), 1–5.

Carthey, J., Walker, S., Deelchand, V., Vincent, C. and Harrop, V. (2011), Breaking the rules: Understanding non-compliance with policies and guidelines, *British Medical Journal*, 343, 5283.

Chen, L. (2019), A review of research on whistle-blowing, *American Journal of Industrial and Business Management*, 9, 295–305.

Chudasama, D. (2021), Why do you need a leader instead of a boss to succeed? *Nolegein Journal of Leadership and Strategic Management*, 4 (1), 24–29.

Cleary, M. and Lees, D. (2019), The role of conscience in nursing practice, *Issues in Mental Health Nursing*, 40 (3), 281–283.

Collins, A. and Cartwright, S. (2012), Why come to work ill? Individual organizational factors underlying presenteeism, *Employee Relations*, 34 (4), 429–442.

Dulon, M., Stranzinger, J., Wendeler, D. and Nienhaus, A. (2020), Causes of needlestick and shaps injuries when using devices with and without safety features, *International Journal of Environmental Research and Public Health*, 17, 8721.

Elliott, P. (2013), Moving from clinical supervision to person-centred development: A paradigm change, in Jasper, M., Rosser, M. and Mooney, G. (eds.), *Professional Development, Reflection and Decision-Making in Nursing and Health Care*, Chichester, Wiley Blackwell, 171.

Elliott, P., Storr, J. and Jeanes, A. (2016), *Infection Prevention and Control*, Boca Raton, Taylor and Francis Group, 63–77.

Festinger, L. (1962), Cognitive dissonance, *Scientific American*, 207, 93–102.

Goodman, J. (1984), Reflection and teacher education: A case study and theoretical analysis, inter-changes, in Jasper, M. (2003 ed.), *Beginning Reflective Practice*, Cheltenham, Nelson Thornes, 72–76.

Grimmond, T., Sunley, K., Gallagher, R., Harrison, R., Oorthuysen-Dunne, J. and Chappell, W. (2020), *Blood and Body Fluid Exposures in 2020*, London, Royal College of Nursing.

Hayward, R. (2012), The invention of the psychosocial: An introduction, *History of the Human Sciences*, 25 (95), 3–12.

Hussein, D. and Saad, W. (2021), Prevalence of sharps injuries among nursing staff at hospitals in Kirkuk, city, *Kufa Journal for Nursing Sciences*, 10 (2).

Ion, R., Jones, A. and Craven, R. (2016), Raising concerns and reporting poor care in practice, *Nursing Standard*, 31 (15), 55–62.

Kinman, G. (2019), Sickness presenteeism at work: Prevalence, costs and management, *British Medical Bulletin*, 129, 69–78.

Lawton, R. and Parker, D. (2002), Judgements of the rule-related behaviour of health care professionals: An experimental study, *British Journal of Health Psychology*, 7, 253–265.

Maxwell, E. (2017), Good leadership in nursing: What is the most effective approach? *Nursing Times*, 113 (9), 18–21.

McLeod, S. (2016), Id, ego and superego, simple psychology, Available Online at: https://cpb-ca-c1.wpmucdn.com/myriverside.sd43.bc.ca/dist/b/55/files/2017/10/simplypsychology.org-psyche-10czxts.pdf#:~:text=According%20to%20Freud%27s%20model%20of%20the%20psyche%2C%20the,between%20thedesires%20of%20the%20id%20and%20the%20super-ego Accessed: 28 July 2022.

Medical and Legal Concepts LLC (2016), Nursing nuggets, Available Online at: https://medicale-galconcepts.com/wp-content/uploads/2016/06/NursingNuggets.pdf Accessed: 28 July 2022.

Mekonnen, T., Tefera, M. and Melsew, Y. (2018), Sick at work: Prevalence and determinants among healthcare workers, western Ethiopia: An institution based cross-sectional study, *Annals of Occupational and Environmental Medicine*, 30 (1), 2.

Mlambo, M., Silén, C. and McGrath, C. (2021), Lifelong learning and nurses' continuing professional development, a metasynthesis of the literature. *BMC Nursing*, 20 (1), 62.

Muti'ah, T. (2010), The view of Freud's pleasure principle and the simple hedonism of human being, *Journal Spirits*, 1 (1), Available Online at: www.psikologi.ustjogja.ac.id/wp-content/uploads/2016/02/6_TheViewOfFreudPleasurePrinciplesAndTheSimpleHedonismOfHuman Being_Titik_OK.pdf Accessed: 28 July 2022.

Meyer, H. and Kirsten, T. (2014), The effect of psychological violence in the workplace on health: A holistic eco-system approach, *Journal of Interdisciplinary Health Sciences*, 19 (1), 757–768.

Okuyama, A., Wagner, C. and Bijnen, B. (2014), Speaking up for patient safety by hospital-based health care professionals: A literature review, *BMC Health Services Research*, 14 (61), 1–8.

Oliver, S. (2006), Leadership in health care, *Musculoskeletal Care*, 4 (1), 38–47.

Owen, L., Apps, L., Stanulewicz, N., Hall, A. and Laird, K. (2021), Health care worker knowledge and attitudes towards uniform laundering during the COVID-19 pandemic, *American Journal of Infection Control*, 1–11.

Reason, J., Parker, D. and Lawton, R. (1998), Organizational controls and safety: The varieties of rule-related behaviour, *Journal of Occupational and Organizational Psychology*, 71, 289–304.

Rodrigo-Rincon, I., Irigoyen-Aristorena, I, Tirapu-Leon, B., Zaballos-Barcala, O., Sarobe-Carricas, M., Antelo-Caamaño, M., Lobo-Palanco, J. and Martin-Vizcaino, M. (2022), Do patients and relatives have different dispositions when challenging healthcare professionals about patient safety? Results before and after an educational program, *Journal of Patient Safety*, 8 (1), e45–e50.

Roth, I. and Firsby, J. (1992), *Perception and Representation: A Cognitive Approach*, Buckingham, Open University Press, 18–23.

Smith, L. and Mee, S. (2017), Patient advocacy: Breaking down barriers and challenging decisions, *Nursing Times*, 113 (1), 54–56.

Taylor, S., Butts, M., Cole, M. and Pounds, T. (2021), Are you sick? Understanding the effects of coworker presenteeism on workplace mistreatment, *American Psychological Association*, 106 (9), 1299–1313.

United Nations (1948), *Universal Declaration of Human Rights*, General Assembly Resolution 217A, Available Online at: www.un-documents.net/a3r217a.htm Accessed: 28 July 2022.

Vahdat, S., Hamzehgardeshi, L., Hessam, S. and Hamzehgardeshi, Z. (2014), Patient involvement in health care decision making: A review, *Iranian Red Crescent Medical Journal*, 16 (1), e12454.

Wain, A. (2017), Learning through reflection, *British Journal of Midwifery*, 25 (10), 662–666.

Weinstein, N. (1982), Unrealistic optimism about susceptibility to health problems, *Journal of Behavioural Medicine*, 5, 441–460.

West, M., Armit, K., Loewenthal, L., Eckert, R., West, T. and Lee, A. (2015), *Leadership and Leadership Development in Health Care: The Evidence Base*, London, Faculty of Medical Leadership, The King's Fund Centre for Creative Leadership.

Wigglesworth, N. (2019), Infection control 3: Use of disposable gloves and aprons, *Nursing Times*, 115 (7), 34–36.

Wong, B. and Ginsburg, S. (2017), Speaking up against unsafe unprofessional behaviours: The difficulty in knowing when and how, *British Medical Journal (Quality and Safety)*, 26, 859–862.

WHO (2020), *Core Competencies for Infection Prevention and Control Professionals*, Geneva, World Health Organization.

The Concept of Truth 3

Paul Elliott

Contents

3.1 INTRODUCTION

This chapter is a personal reflection on the concept of truth and its relationship to IPC. In doing this, I will offer various perspectives and examples with the intention of generating reflective thinking and discussion. However, in undertaking to do so, I have not set out to change the world with regards to the concept of truth but rather to offer a few perspectives. The first thought I would offer is, what is truth? The reality of such a statement is that truth can take differing forms (Buzar et al. 2010; Niskanen 2014)—it is personal. List 3.1 offers examples related to the concept of truth.

LIST 3.1 EXAMPLES OF THE MANY FORMS TRUTH CAN TAKE

- Holding of a belief can constitute truth for some based upon an individual's perception of reality (Poslajko 2021). For example, developing such a belief from what an individual hears and sees in the media about a particular person. Such beliefs can emanate from a religious perspective, a culture within which the individual perceives themselves to be a part of, ethnic origin, and individual beliefs established within childhood and adolescence or beliefs that relate to what an individual perceives as relating to their survival, whether that be physical, psychological or social.
- Attitudes can generally be perceived as being connected to a person, a place or an object, which can constitute self-defining truths for an individual (Zunick

et al. 2017). For example, an attitude about another individual or group of individuals irrespective of whether they have met them or not; a place or location such as a city or country irrespective of whether or not the individual has actually been there or not; the beliefs an individual holds related to a given object whether it be in the form of a desire, a past experience or the result of a given need whether that need be physical, psychological or social in its origin.

- In the context of a conspiracy theory (Van Prooijen and Van Vugt 2018), an individual may regard something as constituting truth irrespective of whether or not it constitutes reality in the mind of the individual or is related to an actual event that has occurred. For example, where a conspiracy emanates from the individual's mental state, where an individual is seeking to lessen uncertainty about a given theory or alleged fact as a means of confirming an individual's prejudices or biases or as a means of filling in the gaps of an individual's understanding/lack of understanding regarding an occurrence.
- Truth can be related to an individual's experience at a given moment in time. For example, what is referred to as eyewitness testimony (Manning and Loftus 1996; Ferris et al. 2017) where after observing an event the individual may, for example, be adamant that an object was one colour when it was a completely different colour. Within this context, where time has passed, the individual's memory may have lapsed in terms of being able to remember exactly what took place and as such will unconsciously fill in the gaps, leading to prevarication with regards to what they observed.
- Despite the fact truth may be illusory in nature (De Keersmaecker et al. 2019), it can still be perceived as constituting reality for an individual. For example, the more an untruth is repeated, the more likely it is that people will start to accept it as a truth. It may be gender related in respect of how experiences are interpreted. It may be generational in nature with regards to what is perceived as truth. It may be authoritarian in nature in that it is perceived as being related to position or rank.
- What constitutes truth can be related to what individuals have been told by others and particularly within the context of enhancing aspects of professional practice (McKenna 1997; Eggins and Slade 2015; Merten et al. 2017), including IPC. For example, where one individual is passing information to one or more individuals and because of the position and perceived competence of the individual giving the information, it is perceived as being true.
- An individual's truth can be related to how they perceive themselves, which may be different to how others perceive them (Martin 2014). For example, one individual may perceive that they are behaving appropriately, where others perceive such behaviour differently.
- On meeting another person for the first time, an individual might perceive them based upon their application of stereotypes or an interpretation of body language, but as they get to know this person, they realise that they were mistaken.

The reality of truth is that at an individual level, it lies within the scope of what they wish to perceive constitutes truth. However, there are also socially constructed truths which relate to society (Galbin 2014). Societies may hold different perceptions of what constitutes truth (Choi et al. 2011). The concept of truth can also change over time. There are a range of theories and processes that can serve to impact upon the perception of truth, the degree to which truth is perceived to be so, and the manner in which truth is portrayed. Many of these were presented in Chapter 1 and in List 3.2.

LIST 3.2 THEORIES THAT MAY IMPACT UPON TRUTH RELATED TO PERCEPTIONS AND SUBSEQUENT BEHAVIOUR

- Cognitive Dissonance Theory: If an individual believes or wants to believe something is true, then they will be likely to generate rationalised reasons/ excuses to support their belief (Elliott 2009). In IPC what the practitioner perceives as constituting truth may lead to either safe or unsafe implementation of appropriate IPC practices.
- Unrealistic Optimism Theory: An individual's beliefs regarding their susceptibility or risk of contracting an illness or disease as a result of their health-related behaviours (Ogden 2019). This can be related to the COVID-19 pandemic where despite the evidence and public health messaging, some individuals were unrealistically optimistic about their susceptibility to the virus, and this impacted upon vaccination uptake (Gassen et al. 2021; Fisk 2021; Alemayehu et al. 2022).
- Cognitive Economy Theory: A lack of perspective can allow an individual to perceive what they wish by failing to look beyond the obvious and failing to take a broader perspective. The practitioner who allows themselves to become cognitively economic in relation to the practice will become task orientated, unidirectional in the interventions they make and the way in which they adhere to evidence-based practices.
- Protection Motivation Theory: Individuals need to believe that by cognitively assessing the severity or susceptibility to given behaviours (Ogden 2019), they will be able to make a choice as to whether such a behaviour will be safe for them to carry out. Whatever the individuals conclude for them, it will constitute truth. This can impact on a health worker's adherence to personal protective equipment, as detailed in standard precautions (List 3.3).

LIST 3.3 ELEMENTS OF THE PROTECTION MOTIVATION THEORY RELATED TO THE USE OF STANDARD PRECAUTIONS

3.3 A:

1. The potential outcome severity of not applying the correct precautions.
2. The level of perceived susceptibility to contracting an infection influences the practitioner's application of the correct precautions.

3. The degree to which their responsive effectiveness of their intervention would be if the practitioner did not adopt the appropriate precautions.
4. Where self-efficacy is concerned the practitioner would reflect upon their beliefs in relation to their ability to complete their intervention and their ability to complete a particular task without exposing themselves to the risk of cross infection.
5. The level of fear and anxiety the practitioner is experiencing would serve to impact upon whether or not they wished to undertake the intervention.

Extracts from Ogden (2019)

The practitioner will establish behavioural intentions relating to what they propose to do and within that context will hold the belief that the decision they make will constitute truth. However, this presents a somewhat negative perspective except for self-efficacy. A more positive and modified approach is listed in 3.3B, the positive motivational outcome perspective relating to PPE usage.

LIST 3.3 THE POSITIVE MOTIVATIONAL OUTCOME PERSPECTIVE

3.3 B:

1. Reward—adopting the appropriate standard precautions will lead to the practitioner feeling a sense of reward for an intervention well done.
2. Protection—wearing the appropriate PPE according to standard precautions will lead to the practitioner knowing that they will have attempted to safeguard both the individual and themselves from the potential of cross infection.
3. Receptive—wearing the appropriate PPE, they will have been sensitive to the individual's needs in terms of protecting them from any potential risk of cross infection from the practitioner.
4. Person centredness—wearing of appropriate PPE will demonstrate the principle of to do no harm and to be person centred in undertaking the intervention.
5. Composed—where the practitioner understands they have the knowledge, skills and appropriate attitudes that will facilitate them in easing any anxiety the individual might be experiencing through the process of effective communication and reassurance within the context of article 10 of the Human Rights Act (Wilkinson and Caulfield 2001).

In offering this alternative perspective, the practitioner will establish behavioural intentions as to what they will do, which will, to the practitioner, constitute a truth.

- Biopsychosocial Theory: This theory is aligned to the biomedical model (Wade and Halligan 2004). In person-centred care, the biomedical model is considered outdated, outmoded, and its application within any aspect of health or social care practice may be considered unsafe. Not least is the unidirectional way it perceives an individual only from a physical/physiological needs standpoint.

Although this model may acknowledge the existence of an individual's psychological and social needs, it considers them to be non-essential (Lane 2014). The biomedical model has been criticised because it fails to offer a truthful perspective of an individual with a health or social care problem or need.

In contrast to the biomedical model is the biopsychosocial model, which emanated from Engle's (1977, 1980) original theory where he attempted to incorporate the psychological and social needs of an individual with those of the physical/physiological needs. Although the biopsychosocial model has been criticised, many perceive it as being a central aspect of health and social care provision in demonstrating enhanced professional practice, improved health outcomes, which may also have the potential to increase recovery times (Taukeni 2020). Consequently, holistic interventions and care acknowledges that the biopsychosocial model constitutes a truthful alternative to the biomedical model.

- Correspondence Theory: Ingthorsson (2019) recognises that different theorists approach the question of truth from differing perspectives. As there are multiple theories/approaches related to the concept of truth, and as these theories are held to be true, it might also be postulated that truth is relative to reality. However, who's reality are we speaking of? The reality of the individual practitioner or the realities of others? Schutz (1945) identified that the origin of all reality is subjective, and anything which comes to an individual's attention will constitute reality for them, summarised nicely in the phrase "perception is reality." As such, it might be further postulated that one individual's reality is as true as any other individual's reality. For example, within a clinical practice context, a practitioner may not be cognisant of the multiple risks posed by microbes because microbes are invisible. Yet from the practitioner's perspective, this is based upon what they perceive to be true. Support for this can be exemplified with regards to the process of cognitive economy and unrealistic optimism (Elliott 2009).

- Consensus Theory: In this approach, if sufficient individuals agree or reach a consensus (Neves 2015) about something, it may be accepted as true through consensus. However, such a consensus does not necessarily constitute truth but can simply be a subjective perspective held by, for example, a group of individuals. There are examples of this in organisations, conferences, and colloquium though consensus changes and does not guarantee safe or ethical practice.

The concept of truth and IPC manifests in a range of misconceptions and fallacies (Elliott et al. 2016). List 3.4 outlines some of these.

LIST 3.4 MISCONCEPTIONS AND FALLACIES RELATED TO IPC

- *This disease is irrelevant to me as I have been inoculated!* The problem with this belief is that irrespective of whether an individual has been inoculated, there can still be the potential for a given disease to be contracted.

- *Cleansing of the hands is not necessary if I have been wearing gloves!* There are multiple problems with this belief, including that wearing gloves does not guarantee sufficient protection against contamination and can be subject to damage whilst wearing them.
- *Only those educated to a certain level on IPC understand IPC because they are the experts!* The problem with this belief is that it is not consistent with the principles of lifelong learning. Individuals throughout their lifespan develop many forms of knowledge/skills which serve to provide them with differing types of expertise, and when such is linked to Gardner's theory of multiple intelligences (Gardner and Walters 1993), each type of expertise would be consistent with a given intelligence. Thus, it can be postulated that no one ever becomes an expert.
- *All cleansing solutions, disinfectants, detergents, and sanitisers are alike and equal in their effect!* The problem with this belief is that this is simply not the case. In effect, such beliefs are potentially dangerous and harmful to not only the individual but to others as well whose learning is facilitated by those who promote such beliefs.
- *I have no need to read the IPC policy as I have worked here for so long that I know about infection control!* The problem with this belief is that policies should be reviewed and updated on a regular basis, and as such, changes to the policy will be included based upon the most recent evidence/research findings.
- *Because of staff and equipment shortages, I always simply wash my gloves between different tasks as opposed to changing my gloves every time I should!* The problem with this belief, whether it be related to staffing or lack of equipment, does not detract from the fact that by failing to change gloves as indicated, this constitutes an increased risk of transmission of microbes. Thus, such a belief constitutes a cognitively economic and dangerous approach to the safety of others.

All the cognitively economic beliefs in the previous section have two things in common. First, they are the result of a dissonance-based rationalisation that allows the practitioner to generate a reason related to why their belief is correct. Second, the practitioner has become unrealistically optimistic with regards to the value of such a belief in respect of the safety of others and to themselves.

However, at this point, let us return to the original question, what is truth? Kostenberger (2005) identifies that it is difficult to imagine a more profound question, which has its origins in Greek philosophy, Roman theorising and in the ancient Hebrew, where the concept of truth has its origins in the ancient world. Yet even today the concept of truth remains in many respects a perplexing paradox for us all. For example, truth could be argued to be anything that can be constructed within the mind/imagination of a given individual irrespective of whether it is construed by others to be absurd, illogical, fanciful, a contradiction in terms, ridiculous or simply perceived as a lie. Therefore, truth for one may be puzzling and inconsistent to others. However, just because an individual believes a thing to be true does not make it so! As Russell (1912) identifies where truth is concerned, we must consider a number of themes which are presented within List 3.5.

LIST 3.5 THEMES RELATED TO TRUTH

- There must be an acknowledgement of an opposite or that a given truth is false. We cannot simply accept that truth is a one-way process because if this were the case, there would be no opportunity to challenge such and that every truth would be factual.
- It must be predisposed to something that is factual. However, where a thing is perceived as being factual, it does not follow that it constitutes truth. Let us consider this within the context of two things:
  1. History is largely based on information and writings from the past. However, just because something historical has been written down, it does not necessarily constitute truth. What an individual perceives to be true and subsequently records reflects their perspective of a given event, which in turn would be based upon their subjective perceptions. Historical truth is based on the records of the victorious and powerful, not the oppressed or defeated, and may not offer an objective view. People's subjective perceptions have been found to be questionable (Lupyan 2017).
  2. Science/research provides us with information which is perceived as constituting truth. However, not all the findings of science/research constitute truth, and Loannidis (2005), Vaux (2016) and Nurunnabi and Hossain (2019) all indicate that falsification and plagiarism of data occur in relation to published materials on more occasions than one might imagine.

Zolkefu (2018) postulates, within the context of health professional practice, being truthful is to do the right thing but asks if lying can also be acceptable if it saves a life. Within the context of article 2 of the Human Rights Act (Wilkinson and Caulfield 2001) argues that undertaking to lie would seem to have value. However, this then presents an ethical dilemma in relation to each profession's code of professional conduct/practice. To what extent should we tell the truth? For example, within the context of IPC and the undertaking of hand hygiene prior to undertaking an intervention—would you as a practitioner who has not undertaken such a process be honest and truthful to another individual if asked? In this regard, I invite you to consider the reflection exercises 3.1 and 3.2 in the next section.

3.2 REFLECTION EXERCISE 3.1: YOURSELF

Consider the following questions and contemplate what your truthful response might be:

- If you had omitted hand hygiene for whatever reason and were then asked by a colleague, would you acknowledge to the individual that you had done so?
- Would you evade or avoid answering the question?
- Would you tell an untruth so as not to cause them anxiety or stress?

- Would you simply not communicate with the individual and ignore what they have asked?
- Would you go and immediately perform hand hygiene if it were indicated?

3.3 REFLECTION EXERCISE 3.2: A COLLEAGUE

Consider the following questions and contemplate what your truthful response might be:

- If a colleague had omitted hand hygiene for whatever reason at a critical moment, would you approach the practitioner irrespective of who they were and bring this to their attention?
- If it were a practitioner who was senior to you, would you approach them and bring this to their attention?
- If it were a practitioner who could influence your future career, would you approach them and bring this to their attention?
- Would you simply ignore the fact that you are aware of the practitioner's failure to undertake hand hygiene, say nothing and let them continue with their IPC practice knowing this may contribute to a future infection?
- Would you wait until after they had carried out whatever it was they were intending to undertake and then raise the matter with them?

Having undertaken both reflection exercises, consider your responses and reflect upon, if any, similarities or differences were either consistent, professional or unprofessional.

In this chapter I have attempted to offer a variety of perspective related to the concept of truth and its relationship to aspects of IPC. Hopefully it will serve to facilitate you towards contemplating further the concept of truth and perhaps reflection upon these questions: Who knows? Who cares?

3.4 REFERENCES

Alemayehu, A., Yusuf, M., Demissie, A. and Abdullahi, Y. (2022), Determinants of Covid-19 vaccine uptake and barriers to be vaccinated among first-round eligible for Covid-19 vaccination in Eastern Ethiopia: A community based cross-sectional study, *SAGE Open Medicine*, 10, 1–9.

Buzar, S., Jalsenjak, B., Krkac, K., Lukin, J., Mladic, D. and Spajic, I. (2010), Habitual lying, *Philosophical Papers and Reviews*, 2 (3), 34–39.

Choi, H., Park, H. and Oh J. (2011), Cultural differences in how individuals explain their lying and truth-telling tendencies, *International Journal of Intercultural Relations*, 35, 749–766.

De keersmaecker, J., Dunning, D., Pennycook, G., Rand, D., Sanchez, C., Unkelbach, C. and Roets, A. (2019), Investigating the robustness of the illusory truth effect across individual differences in cognitive ability, need for cognitive-closure, and cognitive style, *Personality and Social Psychology Bulletin*, 46 (2), 204–215.

Eggins, S. and Slade, D. (2015), Communication in clinical handover: Improving the safety and quality of the patient experience, *Journal of Public Health Research*, 4, 17 (3), 197–199.

Elliott, P. (2009), *Infection Control: A Psychosocial Approach to Changing Practice*, Boca Raton, Taylor and Francis, 73–99.

Elliott, P., Storr, J. and Jeanes, A. (2016). *Infection Prevention and Control: Perceptions and Perspectives*, Boca Raton, Taylor and Francis.

Engle, G. (1977), The need for a new medical model: A challenge for biomedicine, *Science*, 196, 129–135.

Engle, G. (1980), The clinical application of the biopsychosocial model, *American Journal of Psychiatry*, 137, 535–544.

Ferris, K., Bond-Fraser, L. and Fraser, I. (2017), Eyewitness testimony: Assessing the knowledge and beliefs of students studying policing, *International Journal of Liberal Arts and Social Science*, 5 (2), 32–47.

Fisk, R. (2021), Barriers to vaccination for coronavirus disease 2019 (Covid-19) control: Experience from the United States, *Global Health Journal*, 5 (1), 51–55.

Galbin, A. (2014), An introduction to social constructionism, *Social Research Reports*, 26, 82–92.

Gardner, H. and Walters, J. (1993), *Questions and Answers about Multiple Intelligences Theory, Multiple Intelligences: The Theory in Practice*, New York, Basic Books, 35–48.

Gassen, J., Nowak, T., Henderson, A., Weaver, S., Baker, E. and Muehlenbein, M. (2021), Unrealistic optimism and risk for Covid- 19 disease, *Frontiers in Psychology*, 12, 1–16.

Heidegger, M. (1998), Plato's doctrine of truth, Available Online at: http://artsingames.free.fr/Heidegger,%20Martin%20-%20Plato's%20Doctrine%20of%20Truth.pdf   Accessed: 28 July 2022.

Ingthorsson, R. (2019), There's no truth-theory like the correspondence theory, *Discusiones Filosoficas*, 20 (34), 25–41.

Kostenberger, A. (2005), "What is truth?" Pilate's question in its larger biblical context, *Journal of the Evangelical Theological Society*, 48, 33–62.

Lane, R. (2014), Is it possible to bridge the biopsychosocial and biomedical models? *BioPsychoSocial Medicine*, 8 (3).

Loannidis, J. (2005), Why most published research findings are false, *PloS Medicine*, 2 (8), 0696–0701.

Lupyan, G. (2017), How reliable is perception? *Philosophical Topics*, 45 (1), 81–106.

Manning, C. and Loftus, E. (1996), Eyewitness testimony and memory distortion, *Japanese Psychological Research*, 38 (1), 5–13.

Martin, S. (2014), Human perception: A comparative study of how others perceive me and how I perceive myself, Available Online at: www.diva-portal.org/smash/get/diva2:799043/FULLTEXT01.pdf Accessed: 28 July 2022.

McKenna, L. (1997), Improving the nursing handover report, *Professional Nurse*, 12 (9), 637–639.

Merten, H., van Galen, L. and Wagner, C. (2017), Safe handover, *British Medical Journal*, 359, 4328.

Neves, M. (2015), Consensus, in Have, H. (ed.), *Encyclopaedia of Global Bioethics*, Berlin, Springer Science, 1–9.

Niskanen, V. (2014), Prospects for truth valuation in fuzzy extended logic, in Koczy, L., Pozna, C. and Kacprzyk, J. (eds.), *Issues and Challenges of Intelligent Systems and Computational Intelligence*, London, Springer, 3–13.

Nurunnabi, M. and Hossain, M. (2019), Data falsification and question on academic integrity, *Accountability in Research Policies and Quality Assurance*, 26, 108–122.

Ogden, J. (2019), *Health Psychology* (6th ed.), London, McGraw Hill, 5–10, 31 and 38–39.

Poslajko, K. (2021), How to think about the debate over the reality of beliefs, *Review of Philosophy and Psychology*, Available Online at: https://doi.org/10.1007/s13164-021-00551-8 Accessed: 28 July 2022.

Russell, B. (1912), *"What is Truth?" in Problems of Philosophy*, Oxford, Oxford University Press, Available Online at: https://philosophy.lander.edu/intro/articles/correspondence-a.pdf Accessed: 28 July 2022.

Schutz, A. (1945), On multiple realities, *Philosophy and Phenomenological Research*, 5 (4), 533–576.

Taukeni, S. (2020), Biopsychosocial model of health, *Psychology and Psychiatry*, 4 (1).

van Prooijen, J. and van Vugt, M. (2018), Conspiracy theories: Evolved functions and psychological mechanisms, *Perspectives on Psychological Science*, 13 (6), 770–788.

Vaux, D. (2016), Scientific mis conduct: Falsification, fabrication, and misappropriation of credit, in Bretag, T. (ed.), *Handbook of Academic Integrity*, Singapore, Springer, 895–911.

Wade, D. and Halligan, P. (2004), Do biomedical models of illness make for good healthcare systems? *British Medical Journal*, 329, 1398–1401.

Wilkinson, R. and Caulfield, H. (2001), *The Human Rights Act: A Practical Guide for Nurses*, London, Whurr, 23–43.

Zolkefli, Y. (2018), The ethics of truth-telling in health-care settings, *The Malaysian Journal of Medical Sciences*, 25 (3), 135–139.

Zunick, P., Teeny, J. and Fazio, R. (2017), Are some attitudes more self-defining that others? Assessing self-related attitude functions and their consequences, *Personality and Social Psychology Bulletin*, 43 (8), 1136–1149.

PART 2

Leadership Perspectives

Leadership and Influence in Infection Prevention and Control

4

Julie Storr

Contents

If the top is not interested, it will not happen.

(Koegler 2011)

4.1 INTRODUCTION

Leadership is well recognised as a prerequisite for successful implementation of (what are often complex) IPC practices and interventions, related ultimately to improving the quality of health service delivery and the outcomes of those receiving care (WHO 2020). Leadership and a supportive culture have been described as the foundation that supports the implementation and sustainability of proven interventions and practices to ensure quality (WHO et al. 2018). Traditional approaches to leadership have tended to focus on developing individual capacity at the expense of developing collective capability or embedding the development of leaders within the context of the organisation in which they work (West et al. 2014). Leadership and influence are both relevant and critically important now and in the future for all those who have a stake in making IPC work. The relationship between leadership and communication, including risk communication, is key

DOI: 10.1201/9781003379393-6

since the need to convince others of the value of IPC measures is an important part of the role and competence of an IPC leader.

BOX 4.1   REFLECTIONS ON IPC LEADERSHIP

Before reading on, consider how IPC is perceived in your area of work. Would you say it is generally positive? Do you think that the IPC team are respected by different professional groups in the organisations in which you work? Away from the work environment, do you think the media portrays IPC in the best light (think for example about how television and film portrays outbreaks of infection in health care)? Have you ever explored how IPC-related issues are presented and addressed across social media? What do you think can be done to influence all this?

4.2 A PERSONAL PERSPECTIVE ON LEADERSHIP AND IPC

Looking back to the last century, one of the key recommendations from my masters of business administration (MBA) dissertation (Storr 2001) was the need to strengthen how we talk about IPC and the need to develop marketing plans, both in hospitals and nationally, to enhance the strategic impact and influence of IPC leaders. The MBA was stimulated by a personal interest in the subject of strategy and leadership within IPC, particularly how IPC individuals and teams were perceived by managers and leaders within the English NHS. There was an acknowledgement at that time that senior management were not always engaged in IPC and that their understanding of the depth and breadth of the speciality was limited. Interviews with executive level leaders revealed interesting findings, including seeing IPC as an "orphan service which free-floats within the organisation and is not very main stream." Most leaders only took notice of IPC during an outbreak. At that time, the dissertation described the inability to demonstrate value as the "Achilles heel" of IPC teams, and that until such time that IPC is confident of its own contribution, the situation was unlikely to change.

4.3 HISTORY AND NOW

What can we learn from history about IPC leadership and influence? Over the last few decades the influence of local and international outbreaks, notably of MRSA and C difficile (Edgeworth et al. 2020), Ebola virus disease (Coltart et al. 2017) and the increasing focus on the global threat posed by antimicrobial resistance (O'Neil 2016), influenced the specialty of IPC in a number of ways. At the international level, the World Health

Organization (WHO) recognised IPC by establishing a formal IPC programme and developing the first international guidelines on IPC (Storr et al. 2017) and a related set of core competencies (WHO 2020). Both of these have interesting things to say about leadership and strategy. IPC is positioned as critical to safe, quality health care, and for it to be effective requires effective leadership.

Yet anecdotally, as highlighted later in the chapter, there seems to be a lack of IPC influence at the decision-making table in many countries of the world. A recent Cochrane review highlighted the need for clear communication of IPC strategies as fundamental for effective implementation of guidelines (Houghton et al. 2020). IPC is and always has been a social, not purely a technical, discipline. It calls for leadership approaches that embrace the socio adaptive and do not rely on the power that comes with being an expert. IPC has much to learn from exploring the social interactions in which IPC takes place, taking account of the psychology of the organisations in which IPC practitioners work. Too often, the status quo has been one of IPC as enforcer—a member of "the germ police." Looking at how IPC is often addressed across social media by fellow clinicians can make for depressing reading. The example quoted here from a clinical lecturer in 2022 is representative of many I have come across over the last decade: "Will the infection control cult in the NHS ever be remotely evidence based/internally consistent?" Ward (2012) highlighted the negative attitudes towards IPC from qualified staff who perceived IPC measures as an additional workload burden as opposed to an integral aspect of patient safety and quality care. Informed by my own experiences and current discourse with IPC practitioners across many countries, this remains relevant, and in some respects, IPC could be described as a specialty in need of strong, credible leadership.

Closing wards and isolating patients with certain conditions is one accepted part of outbreak management. During the COVID-19 pandemic, restrictions were implemented on a scale not seen before in most people's lifetime. Many who read this book will have experienced restricted access to health and care institutions—"visitors" were forbidden or severely restricted as part of measures to curb the spread of the virus and protect the vulnerable. This particular issue is explored in detail in Chapter 8.

In a pandemic and during other outbreaks, there is an issue of expediency, for example, closing a ward or isolating a patient until the full picture is determined. Sometimes the evidence base changes, and therefore guidelines change rapidly. Sometimes guidance simply isn't followed or people interpret them in the wrong way, fuelled by fear or misguided logic. Sometimes leadership that facilitates and supports implementation of guidance is lacking for many reasons. In some situations, there is little or no evidence, and waiting until there is evidence isn't an option. Think back to the early stages of HIV, of Zika and of course COVID-19. In these instances, leaders had to make decisions and influence others based on expert experience and consultation. One of the problems is that there is rarely consensus when many experts are convened in such emergency situations, and it is in these instances IPC leadership should come to the fore and exert its influence. But IPC needs to be at the table. Without this, the absence of evidence, coupled with expert consensus and often an IPC vacuum opens the door to those with little or no IPC knowledge to erroneously dictate what should happen to prevent germ transmission. What happened with visitor restrictions was that in many cases, they persisted over many months, even years. This reveals much about IPC leadership and influence. In many countries, IPC was not listened to, or at the very least was misunderstood or at worst misapplied—with devastating human consequences. Here, attention is turned to why this might be so. Before reading on, look at the questions in Box 4.2—what do they make you think and feel?

BOX 4.2   QUESTIONS ON LEADERSHIP AND THE IPC TEAM

- Think about the IPC team where you work (if one exists). Who leads the team? Are they visible and approachable to you, to your team, to clinicians and to management?
- Would you describe the leader as strong, credible and influential?
- Where appropriate, what competencies do they possess that result in them perceived as a leader?
- To what extent, if any, do you consider tribalism to be an issue that affects leadership in IPC, for example, between nurses and doctors or between infectious diseases clinicians and virologists and microbiologists?

4.4 MICRO, EVERYDAY LEADERSHIP AND THE POWER OF "WHY"

Chapter 8 explores in depth IPC and compassion and the consequences of inappropriate application or misapplication of IPC measures. This is a strange problem because it is not concerned with the harm caused directly by microbes, rather to the collateral damage of the preventative measures put in place to stop microbes from spreading—what Parker described as the "double iatrogenic effect" (Parker 2011). Stopping this collateral damage requires IPC leadership—not necessarily solely what might be considered conventional leadership, but rather the micro, everyday leadership that is equally important. Although not overt, Chapter 8 also raises many aspects of leadership, and reading this chapter as a companion piece to what is addressed here is highly recommended. In Chapter 8 we learn how, in response to visitor restrictions in long-term care, many people stood up and put their name to an open letter aiming to challenge what was happening, including past, current, and incoming presidents of the Infection Prevention Society of the UK and Ireland. The *Nursing Times* and one of its senior journalists also stepped up and showed leadership by enabling publication of the letter in an open-access format (Storr 2020a). What accompanied this was a deluge of personal messages, emails and tweets from colleagues, from people who had loved ones in care and residential homes, from academics and clinicians in the UK and overseas, all with a common theme—outrage, distress, puzzlement, frustration and pain. Figure 4.1 highlights some of these anonymised messages, summarised here by one such individual: "We (IPC practitioners) are just not being listened to by those

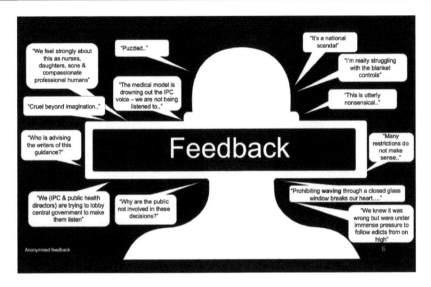

FIGURE 4.1   Anonymised messages from IPC practitioners on visitor restrictions

making the big decisions at the top table." The *Nursing Times* letter highlights the power of collaboration and leadership. It is the antidote to what happens all too quickly in today's social media world, where platforms are used to vent furious rants, fuelled by anger and most likely fear. Rather, what was demonstrated was how working collectively and quickly as a group of committed individuals could develop a set of clear, focused solutions that if acted on immediately would ameliorate harm and suffering to residents and their loved ones. Dixon-Woods (2019) in her essay "How to improve healthcare improvement" reflected that "policy makers would do well to recognise how much more can be achieved through professional coalitions of the willing than through too many imposed, compliance focused diktats."

What can be learned from this example? At the very least, it illustrates that standing up against injustices doesn't need to be riotous. It can involve a single person talking to another person and asking just one simple question—"why?"—"Why can a husband of 50 years not be trusted with the same IPC measures that are being advocated for health workers so that he can sit in a room and hold his wife's hand and comfort her in times of distress?" In laying out how a vision of compassion might be achieved in the English NHS, the then chief nurse talked about the need for leadership at every level, in particular, leadership that champions change and creates an environment where the courage to speak out is welcomed and encouraged (Department of Health and NHS Commissioning Board 2012). This can be manifested by asking "why" by those concerned about IPC recommendations and their impact on the physical and psychosocial wellbeing of people. Asking "why" in this context is probably one of the most powerful words an IPC practitioner or health worker or patient or family member can ever ask. But why itself is not a solution. What is also needed, where appropriate, is action. This is where leadership comes in.

BOX 4.3   LEADERSHIP AND IPC

Before reading on, consider and reflect on the following:

- What exposure have you had so far to leadership development?
- What do you look for in a leader?
- Who is the best leader you have ever worked with and why?
- Have you developed or thought about your own leadership philosophy?

As an IPC practitioner or someone interested in IPC, there are many sources of knowledge and inspiration that can be drawn on to strengthen our role as leaders. This chapter will not replicate what is already out there but it acknowledges that there are courses and textbooks and academic papers that can be consulted by the interested reader. Depending on one's country of work, there will no doubt be a plethora of leadership courses or modules available, some of which will be specific to the IPC practitioner, some more general. It is important to be aware of these.

Leadership theories come in and out of fashion, and caution should be expressed in fixating too much on these, important and useful as they are. There are some insights and themes and words which transcend many of the theories, and these include, for example, leaders need to influence and have a vision and be visible (Frenk 2010). The theories describe different types of leader and leadership styles: situational, transformational, authentic, transactional, compassionate, humble, participatory, distributed, charismatic. The list goes on, but underlying all these are a few assumptions. Based on some recent teachings (Gundlach 2017), here are four of those assumptions. There are many more, and each reader will have their own:

1. Passion is important in leaders, but it should not be mechanistic—it must be authentic.
2. "Felt leadership" is essential—especially in times of uncertainty and change—managing and leading by being visible matters. People should be able to know you, to see you and to feel you. This can really make a difference.
3. Good leaders are good teachers—leaders shape and frame the message and the meaning.
4. The only leadership is ethical leadership—our integrity defines us. Ethics is a social construction concerned with human relationships, matters of justice and duty, responsibility and competence and the greater good. IPC practitioners need to be the ones demonstrating ethical leadership—particularly in times of uncertainty and crisis.

Both the published literature and international guidance in relation to IPC reveals a number of relevant and interesting insights on leadership, including on what is meant by "good leadership." The ability to communicate clearly, effectively and with gravitas, so as to convince others of the need to take certain measures, seems to be a critical skill. Being respected and trusted so that people will follow the advice given by IPC practitioners is also important. All this is reinforced in WHO's core competencies for IPC issued in

2020—leadership and communication skills highlighted as critical to interact with teams and senior management and health workers *per se* and patients and families and other audiences. WHO goes on to state that leaders support others to develop, implement and evaluate their own solutions to problems. A Health Foundation report (2015) emphasised how study participants working in the English NHS focused on the power of strong leadership as necessary for effective organizational IPC. Two views were expressed—one was the need for strong leadership from IPC staff themselves, but importantly, the second emphasised the need for clinicians working on the front line to own and lead IPC themselves. A key lesson from the report was that leadership for IPC needs to be distributed throughout an organisation, with clinical champions identified in all areas. This was found to be important particularly since at the sharp end of care, the report describes the constant competition between immediate priorities and routine best practices. What this interesting report reveals is the need for IPC practitioners to be both strong and influential leaders in their own right but also effective mentors capable of empowering others to own IPC. These two skills require investment in leadership development at the very least.

4.5 WHAT HAPPENS NEXT?

What might IPC practitioners and educators focus on in the future in order to strengthen their leadership and influence? Reflecting on history, including recent personal experiences at the international level, and informed by the literature, the future for IPC leadership holds much promise. Here are some final reflections that might help IPC practitioners better speak truth to power and to influence others moving forward. The collateral damage that has happened throughout history when IPC precautions are implemented in a vacuum, without sufficiently addressing the person on the receiving end of the precautions (and their loved ones), is a lot to do with leadership. It's important with the passage of time that the lessons learned about IPC leadership and influence during pandemic and other times are not forgotten. An excellent piece in *The New Yorker* by Michael Specter written on the back of the Ebola outbreak of 2014/15 is of relevance when we consider what happens next. In it he reflected on our response to pandemics: "First, there is the panic. Then, as the pandemic ebbs, we forget. We can't afford to do either." Reflecting on the COVID-19 pandemic and other global threats, such as the Ebola outbreak of 2015, has generated five leadership lessons that might ensure that many of the harrowing lessons of history are not forgotten.

1. **There is more than one way to do IPC.** IPC is not and should never be solely about the technical, the microbes, and the traditional approaches to investigating and managing these. A depth of understanding of different approaches and complementary (but very unrelated) disciplines is essential. This is happening already but needs to be accelerated—as a discipline, IPC should develop interests beyond the obvious specialty-related ones: psychology, sociology, human factors, behaviour change, to name but a handful. IPC should not trap itself in the microbiology laboratory or focus disproportionately on the controls at the expense of the compassionate implications and impact on people as a result

of imposing controls. Being a technical specialist shouldn't preclude us from gaining insights into the amazing things that the social sciences have to offer, and emerging literature reveals that this is happening. What this means in practice is that we can commit to infusing IPC, including guidance and policies and training with compassion. This will strengthen the specialty for the better and support all those that the specialty exists to serve. As Dixon-Woods reminds us, research shows how the professions can be hugely important institutional forces for good, playing an invaluable role in working as advocates for improvement, creating alliances with patients, providing training and education, contributing expertise and wisdom, coordinating improvement efforts, and giving political voice for problems that need to be solved at the system level. IPC can be part of this.

2. **IPC is not common sense or basic.** IPC leaders of the future will no longer use this type of language that demeans the specialty and gives carte blanch to the uninformed, including politicians, to stand in front of television cameras infantilizing IPC. "IPC is just common sense" gives permission for IPC to be interpreted by anyone in any way they "think" makes sense, because they have been given permission to do so by repeating the misnomer—it's common sense. Using the phrase may also legitimise potentially inhumane practices undertaken in the name of IPC since those without any depth of understanding of IPC think they understand IPC because it's common sense! Calling a moratorium on the use of the phrase has the potential to strengthen the value of IPC.

3. **Evidence-based scientific guidance and compassion are not mutually exclusive**. In fact, the two are aligned and interconnected. As Chapter 7 highlights, the evidence on compassion as a key ingredient of quality care and IPC is solid and growing. IPC leaders have the chance to influence and persuade others on this important matter and to be the compassionate leaders of the future. Compassionate IPC leadership is as important as keeping abreast of the microbial science. Keeping abreast of the scientific literature and the guidance is of course necessary but not sufficient—IPC practitioners should not be blinded by the science. Infuse IPC guidance with compassion.

4. **Power and influence: language matters.** IPC practitioners understand microbial transmission in a way that no other people in health care do. Together with microbiologists and those working in the laboratories, IPC practitioners have studied this and live and breathe it every day. Focus on this as a key strength and source of legitimacy. It should not be turned into a weakness. IPC specialists possess expert power based on this knowledge and competence, and this should be shared effectively using excellent communication. This will require the strategic development of influencing skills. IPC practitioners are influencers. Part of this will involve being comfortable being challenged. This is about competence. The WHO competencies and those of national professional bodies will be a key resource and should be used as part of development. These competencies make it crystal clear that IPC practitioners are leaders and influencers who must be supported in this quest. Depending on your position—look to your superiors and lobby to be developed to your full potential. One practical way to realise this is to consider how you can be developed in your risk

communication. COVID-19 revealed that people made judgements about what IPC practitioners do and don't do, and this was not always a positive experience. IPC practitioners must get better at their communications, they must speak in a language that their target audience understands. They must ensure the message is loud and clear that IPC is an enabler, not a barrier to safe interactions and care. Bottom line—it's the less tangible soft skills around communication and human relations that are key to unlocking the potential of IPC as powerful influencers of the powerful. More on the power of language can be found in Chapter 11.

5. **IPC is an enabler.** IPC is an enabler of safe care and therefore an enabler of compassionate human interactions of the non-technological kind. A focus on IPC as an enabler shifts thinking away from barriers and strengthens the role of IPC practitioners as the leaders and champions of compassionate solutions. In achieving this, we should encourage others to ask the right questions of us and others, and IPC leaders should be recognised and, where necessary, empowered to challenge decision-makers where appropriate.

4.6 NEXT STEPS

Further research is required in multiple countries on the extent to which IPC has a presence at the decision-making level in countries both in peacetime and during emergencies. IPC societies and professional bodies have a potential role in helping to elevate the status, leadership and influence of the profession, including in lobbying for change. IPC must be better listened to in future international outbreaks. A starting point could be the development of a "model" strategic marketing plan for the specialty. If after reading this chapter you agree that the only leadership is ethical leadership, then on a personal level, if not already undertaken, consider developing your own IPC leadership philosophy (Storr 2020b). As Don Berwick states: go quickly, start now—delay is waste (Berwick 2004).

4.7 REFERENCES

Berwick, D. M. (2004). Lessons from developing nations on improving health care. *BMJ* (Clinical research ed.), 328(7448), 1124–1129.

Coltart, C. E., Lindsey, B., Ghinai, I., Johnson, A. M., & Heymann, D. L. (2017). The Ebola outbreak, 2013–2016: Old lessons for new epidemics. *Philosophical Transactions of the Royal Society of London. Series B, Biological Sciences*, 372(1721), 20160297. https://doi.org/10.1098/rstb.2016.0297.

Department of Health and NHS Commissioning Board (2012). Compassion in practice. Nursing, midwifery and care staff: Our vision and strategy. www.england.nhs.uk/wp-content/uploads/2012/12/compassion-in-practice.pdf. Accessed 13 February 2022.

Dixon-Woods, M. (2019). How to improve healthcare improvement-an essay by Mary Dixon-Woods. *BMJ* (Clinical research ed.), 367, l5514.

Edgeworth, J. D., Batra, R., Wulff, J., & Harrison, D. (2020). Reductions in methicillin-resistant staphylococcus aureus, clostridium difficile infection and intensive care unit-acquired bloodstream infection across the United Kingdom following implementation of a national infection control Campaign. *Clinical Infectious Diseases: An Official Publication of the Infectious Diseases Society of America*, 70(12), 2530–2540.

Frenk, J. (2010). The global health system: Strengthening national health systems as the next step for global progress. *PLoS Medicine*, 7(1), e1000089.

Gundlach, A. M. (2017). *Johns Hopkins School of Public Health*. Foundations of Organizational Leadership Masters Course.

Health Foundation (2015). Infection prevention and control: Lessons from acute care in England: Towards a whole health economy approach. www.health.org.uk/publications/infection-prevention-and-control-lessons-from-acute-care-in-england. Accessed 15 November 2021.

Houghton, C., Meskell, P., Delaney, H., Smalle, M., Glenton, C., Booth, A., Chan, X., Devane, D., & Biesty, L. M. (2020). Barriers and facilitators to healthcare workers' adherence with infection prevention and control (IPC) guidelines for respiratory infectious diseases: A rapid qualitative evidence synthesis. *The Cochrane Database of Systematic Reviews*, 4(4), CD013582.

Koegler, E. (2011). *Insights from a National Health Care Quality Improvement Strategy Meeting*. Technical Report. Published for U.S. Agency for International Development (USAID) by the Health Care Improvement Project. Bethesda, MD: University Research Co., LLC.

O'Neil, J. (2016). *Tackling Drug-Resistant Infections Globally: Final Report and Recommendations*. London, UK: Wellcome Trust & HM Government.

Parker, N. (2011). *The Psychological Impact of Nosocomial Infection: A Phenomenological Investigation of Patients' Experiences of Clostridium Difficile*. [Dissertation]. University of Leicester, Leicester.

Storr, J. (2001). *Do Infection Control Services Function Strategically within the NHS?* Dissertation submitted to Oxford Brookes University for the partial fulfilment of the requirements of the Master of Business Administration, December 2001 (unpublished).

Storr, J. (2020a). Open letter: Infection prevention and control should never be at the expense of compassionate care. *Nursing Times*, 16 October 2020. www.nursingtimes.net/opinion/open-letter-infection-prevention-and-control-should-never-be-at-the-expense-of-compassionate-care-16–10–2020/.

Storr, J. (2020b). Perspectives: Go quickly, start now: A personal leadership philosophy. *Journal of Research in Nursing*, 25(4), 393–397.

Storr, J., Twyman, A., Zingg, W., et al. (2017). Core components for effective infection prevention and control programmes: New WHO evidence-based recommendations. *Antimicrob Resist Infect Control*, 6(6).

Ward, D. J. (2012). Attitudes towards infection prevention and control: An interview study with nursing students and nurse mentors. *BMJ Quality & Safety*, 21(4), 301–306.

West, M., Eckert, R., Steward, K., & Pasmore, B. (2014). *Developing Collective Leadership for Health Care*. London: The King's Fund.

WHO (2020). *Core Competencies for Infection Prevention and Control Professionals*. Geneva: World Health Organization.

WHO, Organisation for Economic Co-operation and Development, World Bank (2018). *Delivering Quality Health Services: A Global Imperative for Universal Health Coverage*. Geneva: World Health Organization.

Power and Compliance Within Infection Prevention and Control Practice

5

Annette Jeanes

Contents

> Control leads to compliance; autonomy leads to engagement.
>
> —Daniel H. Pink

DOI: 10.1201/9781003379393-7

5.1 INTRODUCTION

Infection prevention and control (IPC) compliance is primarily related to achieving and sustaining behaviours and practices which aim to reduce the transmission and the consequences of infection. Optimal IPC practice is heavily reliant on the compliance of people with established standards and the support of organisations. Achieving and sustaining compliance is complex and can be difficult, but there is evidence that power can play an important role.

Compliance has been studied widely, and there is a considerable evidence and experience not only in relation to laws and rules but also in relation to controls and change. Whilst compliance is important in all IPC practice, in the past there has been a particular concentration of research into hand hygiene compliance. Achieving consistently high levels of hand hygiene compliance is important but has been difficult to achieve and sustain in many areas of healthcare practice (Kirkland & Craig 2011). The knowledge gained from work to improve this behaviour can be utilised more generally in IPC, including for example isolation of patients, the correct application and use of PPE and adherence to the principles of asepsis.

5.2 POWER

French and Raven (1959) identified six forms of social power which may influence beliefs, attitudes and behaviours of individuals:

- Coercive power
- Reward power
- Legitimate power
- Expert power
- Referent power
- Informational power

These forms of power are linked to leadership, and their impact is dependent on the people, context and conditions. Coercive power can be used to compel individuals to comply and may be associated with disciplinary actions. This may work in some circumstances, but individuals may resist, some may forget, whilst others ignore the threat when confident that there will be no consequence because they are too important or that no one will notice. In reward power, individuals may see the benefit of a reward and improve compliance at least for the short term. However, this may also be a disincentive if it is perceived to be unfair or if the reward does not materialise. The position held by a person may give them legitimate power, but this may be limited to their tenure and is only applicable within the scope of their responsibility. IPC practitioners have expert power, which relates to the knowledge skills and experience of the individual. This may be perceived by others as valuable and the individual practitioner credible and respected. This increases the potential to influence others on their area of expertise as they trust that the expert is likely to know what they are talking about. Although if the IPC expert is not up to date in the specialist topic or assumes they are omniscient in all matters of IPC, this may undermine their credibility and power (Bergstrom & West 2021). Popular and admired people can exert referent power, which can influence how people behave and what choices they make. These people act as role models and opinion influencers, and their effect on behaviour may persist long term. Informational power relates to the control and dispersal of information. Whilst withholding information can limit the knowledge and hamper decisions, providing information can inform choices and increase knowledge. It is also possible to manipulate information to influence choices and, for example, to justify controls.

5.3 LEADERSHIP

Leadership may encompass all the forms of power identified by French and Raven (1959; Raven 1966) and has an important role in compliance with IPC expectations. There are several forms of leadership, and leadership theories shed insights into how some leaders have powers to compel compliance, others influence the practice of others by acting as a role model, offering support and encouragement, educating, informing and enabling.

Leadership support and commitment has been found to be important in improving compliance and supporting improvement efforts in IPC (Doron et al. 2011; Jamal et al. 2012; Kwok et al. 2017). The position and role of the leader is particularly influential when acting as a role model. In a study by Haessler et al. (2012), it was found that the most senior doctor often leads the team on a ward round, and when the first person entering a patient room cleaned their hands, those following were significantly more likely to clean their hands. In addition, the compliance of the senior doctor influenced hand hygiene whatever their order of entering the room. Lankford et al. (2003) found that in the presence of a noncompliant senior HCW, junior staff were less likely to wash their hands. Whilst Farr (2000) suggested that the presence of negative role models stopped others trying to be compliant with IPC guidelines.

Leadership engagement and support are beneficial to IPC initiatives and practice compliance. Leaders may champion work to remove barriers to compliance (Zingg et al. 2015). Leaders have a role in recognising and presenting coherent arguments for changing practices and prioritising the implementation of beneficial improvements. Leadership support may be present because there is compulsion from elsewhere, for example, government, but is in part reliant on leadership recognising imperfections in reported and observed compliance and understanding the implications of inaction.

Leaders may be influenced by other colleagues, motivated individuals, researchers, educators and patient groups who recognise the value of preventing infection. Local champions may also influence leaders. Gillespie et al. (2007) found that local ownership of hand hygiene responsibility was enhanced by the unit leadership and that sustaining compliance improvements was related to strong leadership and the empowerment of patient advocates.

Strong leadership and support of IPC work is important in a crisis but is also crucial in maintaining an emphasis and commitment long term. It is essential to put in place a consistent approach to improving rules and procedures and the working environment, to improve IPC compliance. The legitimate use of power by leaders can improve and sustain IPC compliance by, for example, supporting IPC education, enabling environmental improvements, monitoring compliance, acting as a role model and, when required, mandating compliance.

5.4 SPEAKING TRUTH TO POWER

Listening to the views of others and a readiness to modify or change views is recognised as an important trait of leadership. However, leaders may not be predisposed to listen. An example is a leader who states, "Don't bring me problems just bring solutions." This effectively prevents a discussion of problems and may intimidate the messenger. Other tactics include organisational barriers to prevent or avoid contact such as basing themselves in a distant office with limited access, meeting by appointment only and frequently cancelling due to more important issues or ensuring contact is sanitised and controlled by middle managers, particularly if the feedback is about their performance.

Unfortunately, issues including the lack of opportunity and confidence to speak up and the need to "fit in" (Barrett & Randle 2008) or give a good impression (Curtis et al. 2003) undermine the flow of perceived truth to power. There is substantial benefit of leaders being present, being curious and encouraging the objective review and evaluation of practice and outcomes related to IPC.

5.5 MEASUREMENT OF COMPLIANCE

It has been suggested that the energy and cost required to produce compliance information would be better spent by those with power being visible in clinical areas, supporting good IPC practice and listening to the experience of the patients and staff (Ling & How 2012). This is not always feasible, and to ensure the interest and energy of IPC compliance is sustained, leaders may in part rely on standardised and comparable performance metrics.

IPC-related performance metrics may be unreliable and can give an inaccurate picture of what is happening in practice (Jeanes et al. 2015). Though audit of IPC practice is popular, being observed may increase compliance (Chen et al. 2015), producing inflated results, and the use of established audit tools in the hands of novices may miss significant IPC issues. The reliability and validity of IPC performance metrics is also influenced by the requirement to meet targets, which may lead to a tick box exercise and is of little value in quality improvement (Jeanes et al. 2015)

In IPC, a continuous quality improvement approach with realistic expectations of compliance can identify human factors (Reason 2000) which are barriers to compliance, such as lack of IPC education and inadequate facilities. This alternative to standardised metrics such as hand hygiene compliance or environmental audits ensures energy and resource are focused on areas where improvements are required and highlights issues which require further significant scrutiny and/or investment.

5.6 FACTORS AFFECTING COMPLIANCE

Whilst power has a significant influence on IPC compliance, it is also affected by other factors, including leadership, organisational culture, context, risk perception, education and background, role, motivation, management of noncompliance, being observed, role models, peer pressure, and the environment.

5.7 ORGANISATIONAL CULTURE

The potential for organisational culture to influence IPC compliance has been recognised (De Bono et al. 2014; van Buijtene & Foster 2019), and it has been suggested that a culture change can improve compliance (Clayton & Griffith 2008; Grayson et al. 2008, 2018). Whilst this may be found in organisations which embrace a safety culture (Caris et al. 2017) and include IPC in the quality improvement and learning strategy, van Buijtene and Foster (2019) suggest that a weak and toxic culture may have a negative effect on compliance.

The management strategy and methods adopted by the organisation are an important factor in the response and compliance of employees. Golden (1992) describes four types of responses to organisational compliance expectations:

- Unequivocal adherence
- Strained adherence
- Secret non-adherence
- Overt non-adherence

Within healthcare organisations, it is likely that all these levels of compliance will be present at some point, although individuals will respond differently and sometimes unpredictably. Whilst unequivocal or even strained adherence to IPC guidelines may be helpful, there is also value in understanding why others deviate from expectations. Indeed, it should be recognised that in some areas of IPC practice that the evidence base is thin or perhaps emerging, and there may not be a robust evidence base for guidance (Dancer 2016).

It may be tempting to apply a "top-down" imposed system, but this can result in little ownership or engagement and some resentment. Challenging guidance and suggesting alternatives may be useful in some circumstances but can be disruptive and undermine confidence in the advice given by the IPC team. Non-adherent practices when no effective or safe alternative is available is problematic and should be proactively managed, including providing evidence, reaching consensus, discouraging noncompliance and monitoring practice.

5.8 CONTEXT

Credibility and pragmatism are important in achieving compliance in IPC practice (Gould & Drey 2013). Understanding and considering the context of practice is essential for success, as whilst expectations of compliance are always high, in some situations—for example, disasters, war, poverty and epidemics—it may not be feasible to achieve what is normally expected, and adherence to basic controls may be all that is possible.

Compliance expectations may also be tempered by situations where compliance is hampered by, for example, lack of supplies, facilities, and staff. In these situations, whilst individuals may want to comply with guidance, their compliance is hindered by the circumstances. In such situations, there is a danger that cultural entrapment of noncompliance may develop where poor practice becomes the norm (van Buijtene & Foster 2019) and where practitioners appear to be coping.

5.9 RECOGNITION AND MANAGEMENT OF NONCOMPLIANCE

An embedded tolerance of suboptimal compliance may also be the consequence of a toxic or poorly managed organisation or one which is inward focused and fails to recognise what good IPC looks like. It may also occur in organisations where a culture of deference is prevalent and in which noncompliance of some people or groups is not challenged whilst others are expected to comply. Whatever the cause, not managing noncompliance with IPC guidance will undermine efforts to improve and sustain compliance.

A starting point for those with power is understanding what is possible and what is a minimum expectation of compliance, as setting unrealistic goals is unlikely to be successful. Exhaustion and stress from the efforts to deliver the unachievable will undermine motivation and job satisfaction. Agreeing to a plan with short-, medium- and long-term objectives is a successful standard approach, and the use of frameworks such as the Behaviour Change Wheel (Michie et al. 2011) provides a structure for the interventions required.

A lack of recognition of why compliance is important may be a factor in noncompliance, and therefore it is essential to ensure the evidence, rationale and consequences are clear and targeted at specific audiences. The way the message is formulated and delivered may affect compliance (Taylor 2015). The role, background, experience, education and motivation of the target audience also influence individual compliance. Those in positions of power may expect their subordinates to want to comply to please or to support an organisational achievement of a target. These expectations may in fact alienate some staff, whilst others will attempt to comply, even when they sometimes do not agree with what is expected.

Role models and influencers have a significant role in IPC compliance. Jang et al. (2010) found that for example the attitudes and practices of doctors significantly influenced the hand hygiene of other healthcare workers (HCW). In the past there have been several examples of suboptimal hand hygiene compliance by doctors which has undermined efforts to improve overall compliance in healthcare (Pittet 2001; Whitby et al. 2007; Azim et al. (2016)). Reasons such as workload, lack of knowledge and difficulties accepting behaviour change (Salemi et al. 2002) have been suggested as reasons for doctors' poor compliance with IPC guidance *per se*. However, in the past, applying the same expectations and challenges to this staff group has sometimes been difficult as they were perceived as "special" or "too valuable to lose or upset." The hierarchy and power structures within health care play a role here. Unfortunately, these perceptions and the underpinning hierarchies and cultures are not shared by pathogens, and therefore the same IPC expectations of compliance apply.

Embedded tolerance or ignoring the noncompliance of some staff or individuals impacts the motivation of others to comply, and part of the role of leaders and those with power and influence is to be seen to challenge noncompliance. In the author's experience, this may be nerve-racking but is valuable. Sometimes these individuals have little self-awareness that they are not compliant or assume that no one has noticed. Box 5.1 presents an illustrative example.

BOX 5.1   EXAMPLE OF SELF-AWARENESS (OR LACK OF) OF LEADERS

There had been several complaints about the hand hygiene of a senior clinician. When questioned, the complainants responded that the individual was too senior and too scary to challenge. Subsequently in a private meeting, the senior clinician was informed of the feedback and concerns about a senior clinician. The clinician demanded to know who this was as they would be severely punished no matter who they were. When informed that they were the person concerned, they were devastated and embarrassed that no one had spoken up before as they were not aware of the problem.

Pursuing IPC compliance can at times be exhausting for those responsible and, in some instances, target setting and monitoring can be counterproductive. In response to potentially punitive consequences of noncompliance, some individuals may "turn a blind eye" rather than challenge, whilst others comply as they fear failure. The purpose of compliance can be "lost in translation" as there may be ambiguity about what is required or gaming to achieve target with no real improvement in practice (Jeanes et al. 2015). There is also a danger of compliance without understanding and an inability to adapt and apply underlying principles or logic. Examples include, "We have to clean this (piece of equipment) every shift even when we do not use it anymore," "We have to use a whole sterile pack even though we only need a swab."

5.10 RISKS

The level of perceived risk affects compliance. This not only affects the urgency and preference for IPC compliance, but there is also evidence that individuals often increase compliance when they believe they are in danger (Bjørkheim & Sætrevik 2022). In such circumstances, there may be a low tolerance of noncompliance amongst peers and organisations for a variety of reasons, including personal safety, potential patient harm, reputational damage and financial costs.

It is unusual for the consequence of noncompliance to be evident immediately as infections take time to develop, and many factors affect transmission and acquisition (Van Seventer & Hochberg 2017). This affects the perception of risk and consequently work to increase awareness is required to enhance risk perception. This is explored in more detail by Sax in Chapter 10.

Whilst the potential for danger and risks may increase compliance, this may also create fear and a reluctance of some staff to put themselves at risk. There is also evidence that factors such as context, knowledge and experience make some people more inclined to take risks and push boundaries (Bodemer & Gaissmaier 2015). Consequently, some may seek to work in specialities where there is risk and the autonomy to use their judgement.

5.11 HUMAN FACTORS

Barriers which contribute to suboptimal compliance include lack of information, knowledge and experience, lack of time, high workload, inadequate equipment and fatigue (Reason 2000). Motivation, education, and social norms are also contributory factors (Kretzer & Larson 1998). It is important to understand that sometimes the best IPC practitioner in the universe will have a limited effect when the barriers to compliance are significant. The role of those with power includes a recognition of barriers to compliance and utilisation of opportunities to improve compliance. Simple and effective strategies include ensuring guidance is accessible, simple, unambiguous and supported by managers (Gurses et al. 2008). Others include support of environmental improvements which optimise IPC compliance and investment in IPC training and education for all staff. These should be part of a multi modal strategy to improve compliance and support the challenge of noncompliance. In Chapter 10 Sax provides a detailed outline of human factors.

5.12 CONCLUSION

Those with power cannot achieve IPC compliance alone, and the engagement and participation of others is a prerequisite to implementation and improvement. Often the key leaders in IPC are the resident IPC experts, but the influence and support of the organisation is essential for success. Factors within the environment can both impede and offer opportunities to improve IPC compliance, but leaders and influencers must be aware of constraints and realistic in expectations. Visible and powerful leadership which challenges noncompliance and champions compliance is likely to have considerable success in IPC.

5.13 REFLECTIONS

1. Can you identify some positive and negative experiences you have encountered in giving or receiving feedback in relation to infection control practice?
2. Have you been trained in the delivery of feedback of performance? Was it or could it be useful for you and your colleagues?
3. Are you a credible expert? How do you demonstrate your credibility?

5.14 REFERENCES

Azim S, Juergens C, McLaws ML. An average hand hygiene day for nurses and physicians: The burden is not equal. *American Journal of Infection Control.* 2016;44:777–81.

Barrett R, Randle J. Hand hygiene practices: Nursing students' perceptions. *Journal of Clinical Nursing.* 2008;17:1851–7.

Bergstrom CT, West JD. *Calling bullshit: The art of skepticism in a data-driven world.* Random House Trade Paperbacks; 2021 Apr 20.

Bjørkheim S, Sætrevik B. *Risk of infection and appeal to public benefit increase compliance with infection control measures*; 2022. https://psyarxiv.com/myv4t/download?format=pdf

Bodemer N, Gaissmaier W. *Risk perception.* Sage; 2015.

Caris MG, Kamphuis PG, Dekker M, de Bruijne MC, van Agtmael MA, Vandenbroucke-Grauls CM. Patient safety culture and the ability to improve: A proof of concept study on hand hygiene. *Infection Control & Hospital Epidemiology.* 2017;38:1277–83.

Chen LF, Vander Weg MW, Hofmann DA, Reisinger HS. The Hawthorne effect in infection prevention and epidemiology. *Infection Control & Hospital Epidemiology.* 2015;36:1444–50.

Clayton DA, Griffith CJ. Efficacy of an extended theory of planned behaviour model for predicting caterers' hand hygiene practices. *International Journal of Environmental Health Research.* 2008;18:83–98.

Curtis V, Biran A, Deverell K, Hughes C, Bellamy K, Drasar B. Hygiene in the home: Relating bugs and behaviour. *Social Science & Medicine.* 2003;57:657–72.

Dancer SJ. Infection control: Evidence-based common sense. *Infection, Disease & Health.* 2016;21:147–53.

De Bono S, Heling G, Borg MA. Organizational culture and its implications for infection prevention and control in healthcare institutions. *Journal of Hospital Infection.* 2014;86:1–6.

Doron SI, Kifuji K, Hynes BT, Dunlop D, Lemon T, Hansjosten K, Cheng T, Curley B, Snydman DR, Fairchild DG. A multifaceted approach to education, observation, and feedback in a successful hand hygiene campaign. *The Joint Commission Journal on Quality and Patient Safety.* 2011;37:3–AP3.

Farr BM. Reasons for noncompliance with infection control guidelines. *Infection Control & Hospital Epidemiology*. 2000;21:411–6.

French JR, Raven B, Cartwright D. The bases of social power. *Classics of Organization Theory*. 1959;7:311–20.

Gillespie EE, ten Berk de Boer FJ, Stuart RL, Buist MD, Wilson JM. A sustained reduction in the transmission of methicillin resistant Staphylococcus aureus in an intensive care unit. *Critical Care and Resuscitation*. 2007;9:161–5.

Golden KA. The individual and organizational culture: Strategies for action in highly-ordered contexts. *Journal of Management Studies*. 1992;29:1–21.

Gould D, Drey N. Types of interventions used to improve hand hygiene compliance and prevent healthcare associated infection. *Journal of Infection Prevention*. 2013 May;14(3):88–93.

Grayson ML, Jarvie LJ, Martin R, Johnson PD, Jodoin ME, McMullan C, Gregory RH, Bellis K, Cunnington K, Wilson FL, Quin D. Significant reductions in methicillin-resistant Staphylococcus aureus bacteraemia and clinical isolates associated with a multisite, hand hygiene culture-change program and subsequent successful statewide roll-out. *Medical Journal of Australia*. 2008;188:633–40.

Grayson ML, Stewardson AJ, Russo PL, Ryan KE, Olsen KL, Havers SM, Greig S, Cruickshank M, Australia HH, National hand hygiene initiative. Effects of the Australian national hand hygiene initiative after 8 years on infection control practices, health-care worker education, and clinical outcomes: A longitudinal study. *The Lancet Infectious Diseases*. 2018;18:1269–77.

Gurses, AP, Seidl, K, Vaidya, V. Systems ambiguity and guideline compliance: A qualitative study of how intensive care units follow evidence-based guidelines to reduce healthcare-associated infections. *BMJ Quality & Safety*. 2008;17: 351–9.

Haessler S, Bhagavan A, Kleppel R, Hinchey K, Visintainer P. Getting doctors to clean their hands: Lead the followers. *BMJ Quality & Safety*. 2012;21:499–502.

Jamal A, O'Grady G, Harnett E, Dalton D, Andresen D. Improving hand hygiene in a Paediatric hospital: A multimodal quality improvement approach. *BMJ Quality & Safety*. 2012 Feb 1;21(2):171–6.

Jang TH, Wu S, Kirzner D, Moore C, Youssef G, Tong A, Lourenco J, Stewart RB, McCreight LJ, Green K, McGeer A. Focus group study of hand hygiene practice among healthcare workers in a teaching hospital in Toronto, Canada. *Infection Control & Hospital Epidemiology*. 2010;31:144–50.

Jeanes A, Coen PG, Wilson AP, Drey NS, Gould DJ. Collecting the data but missing the point: Validity of hand hygiene audit data. *Journal of Hospital Infection*. 2015;90:156–62.

Kirkland K, Craig SR. A *Qualitative Analysis of Facilitators and Barriers to Hand Hygiene Improvement at New Hampshire Hospitals during a Statewide Hand Hygiene Campaign*. *Foundation for Healthy Communities*. Foundation for Healthy Communities; 2011 Nov.

Kretzer EK, Larson EL. Behavioral interventions to improve infection control practices. *American Journal of Infection Control*. 1998;26:245–53.

Kwok YL, Harris P, McLaws ML. Social cohesion: The missing factor required for a successful hand hygiene program. *American Journal of Infection Control*. 2017;45:222–7.

Lankford MG, Zembower TR, Trick WE, Hacek DM, Noskin GA, Peterson LR. Influence of role models and hospital design on the hand hygiene of health-care workers. *Emerging Infectious Diseases*. 2003;9:217.

Ling ML, How KB. Impact of a hospital-wide hand hygiene promotion strategy on healthcare-associated infections. *Antimicrobial Resistance and Infection Control*. 2012;1:1–5.

Michie S, Van Stralen MM, West R. The behaviour change wheel: A new method for characterising and designing behaviour change interventions. *Implementation Science*. 2011;6:1–2.

Pittet D. Improving adherence to hand hygiene practice: A multidisciplinary approach. *Emerging Infectious Diseases*. 2001;7:234.

Reason J. Human error: Models and management. *BMJ*. 2000;320:768–70.

Salemi C, Canola MT, Eck EK. Hand washing and physicians: How to get them together. *Infection Control & Hospital Epidemiology*. 2002;23:32–5.

Taylor RE. The role of message strategy in improving hand hygiene compliance rates. *American Journal of Infection Control*. 2015;43:1166–70.

van Buijtene A, Foster D. Does a hospital culture influence adherence to infection prevention and control and rates of healthcare associated infection? A literature review. *Journal of Infection Prevention*. 2019;20:5–17.

Van Seventer JM, Hochberg NS. Principles of infectious diseases: Transmission, diagnosis, prevention, and control. *International Encyclopedia of Public Health*. 2017:22.

Whitby M, Pessoa-Silva CL, McLaws ML, Allegranzi B, Sax H, Larson E, Seto WH, Donaldson L, Pittet D. Behavioural considerations for hand hygiene practices: The basic building blocks. *Journal of Hospital Infection*. 2007;65:1–8.

Zingg W, Holmes A, Dettenkofer M, Goetting T, Secci F, Clack L, Allegranzi B, Magiorakos AP, Pittet D. Hospital organisation, management, and structure for prevention of health-care-associated infection: A systematic review and expert consensus. *The Lancet Infectious Diseases*. 2015;15:212–24.

Patient Safety, Governance, Leadership and Infection Prevention and Control

Helen Hughes

Contents

DOI: 10.1201/9781003379393-8

6.1 INTRODUCTION TO PATIENT SAFETY LEARNING

Patient Safety Learning is a charity and independent voice for improving patient safety. Since its inception in 2019, it acknowledges that despite an increase in patient safety improvement projects in local organisations across the world, there remains a lack of a systematic approach to sharing knowledge and information about what patient safety initiatives and solutions work. It makes the case that we need urgent system-wide change—to design for safety as a core purpose of health and social care. This chapter frames IPC within the broader patient safety agenda and provides insights on the value of a system-wide approach to improvement, including a focus on understanding how people within the system function.

6.2 WHAT IS PATIENT SAFETY?

Patient safety is the absence of preventable harm to a patient during the process of health care and the reduction of risk of unnecessary harm associated with health care to an accepted minimum. The World Health Organization (WHO) Global Patient Safety Action Plan (WHO 2021) defines this as follows:

> A framework of organized activities that creates cultures, processes, procedures, behaviours, technologies and environments in health care that consistently and sustainably lower risks, reduce the occurrence of avoidable harm, make errors less likely and reduce the impact of harm when it does occur.
>
> (WHO 2021)

As a discipline, patient safety has emerged reflecting the evolving complexity in healthcare systems and the resultant rise of avoidable harm. The ambitions of many patient safety programmes are to identify and mitigate hazards and risk and to reduce the impact of error and harm that occur to patients. Infection prevention and control (IPC) is a key field within this discipline, with its focus on providing an evidence-based approach to preventing patients and healthcare professionals from being harmed. Effective IPC is a core element of the wider challenge of avoidable harm in health care.

6.3 TYPES OF ERRORS AND ISSUES THAT CAUSE AVOIDABLE HARM

As a result of the increasing complexity of health care, there are a range of different ways in which avoidable harm can occur. Five examples of the varied ways in which avoidable harm in health care can occur are presented here: diagnostic errors, medication errors, unsafe surgery, healthcare-associated infections (HCAIs) and communication and information errors.

Diagnostic errors can occur in all healthcare settings and broadly fall into three categories. The first concerns delayed diagnosis—where harm is caused because of a condition not being identified at an earlier stage. Incorrect diagnosis happens when the wrong diagnosis is made, and the true cause is discovered later. Finally, missed diagnosis is where a patient's condition is not identified, leading to no treatment taking place.

Patients can be subject to avoidable harm in a range of different errors in parts of the process around medication, including prescription, dosage, route of medication administration and omission. Prescription errors can manifest themselves in a range of different ways, with patients potentially underprescribed or overprescribed medicines for their condition, or receiving a prescription which does not address their health condition and subsequently resulting in deterioration as a result of this. Dosage errors, whether these are missed doses or incorrect doses, can occur in a range of settings, with a substantial proportion of these relating to children due to the complexity of weight-based paediatric dosing (Gonzales 2010). Mistakes in the administration of medicine can also lead to serious harm, such as administering a medicine which should be taken intravenously by the intrathecal route.

Unsafe surgery is concerned with errors occurring during an operation and can result in serious patient harm, with common patient safety issues including retained foreign objects in the patient's body, wrong site surgery, anaesthesia errors, dentification errors resulting in surgery on the wrong patient and surgical fires.

HAIs are one of the most common adverse events in care delivery and a major public health problem with an impact on morbidity, mortality and quality of life (WHO 2016a). Common determinants of HAI include inappropriate use of invasive devices and antibiotics, high-risk diagnostic or therapeutic procedures, immuno-suppression, other severe underlying illnesses and conditions affecting newborns and older people and substandard application of IPC precautions (WHO 2016b). Communication and information errors are concerned with failures or errors in communication between healthcare professionals and patients, or between healthcare professionals themselves during treatment, and can in many cases result in patients being harmed or receiving substandard care.

A common thread running through each of these is the behaviour of people within the health system and all the importance of understanding all the factors that influence this behaviour.

6.4 SCALE OF AVOIDABLE HARM

So how big of a problem is avoidable harm for health care? Avoidable harm is an issue that affects all healthcare systems, with the WHO estimating that it is one of the ten leading causes of death and disability worldwide (WHO 2019). A recent analysis by the G20 Health and Development Partnership suggests that this translates into over 3 million deaths each year (G20 2021). Research studies indicate that on average, one in ten patients is subject to an adverse event while receiving hospital care (WHO 2021). WHO go on to state that in low- and middle-income countries, this figure could be as high as one in four patients.

In addition to the tragic loss of life and long-term impact of patients' health and well-being, there is also a huge financial burden associated with unsafe care. The direct cost of unsafe care in developed countries is estimated at 12.6% of health expenditure (OECD & SPSC 2020). Worldwide, patient safety issues are forecast to cost the global economy by 2022 a staggering $383.7 billion (G20 2021). These figures only focus on the direct costs, however, with studies looking at the wider economic impact suggesting that this could be even higher (Andel et al. 2012).

Avoidable harm also comes with an untold physical and emotional impact on those affected that is much harder to measure. For those directly affected, there may be both physical and psychological discomfort from remedial treatment, longer hospital stays or disability because of avoidable harm, in addition to a diminished trust in the healthcare system and professionals by patients. Meanwhile for healthcare professionals themselves, this can result in a loss of morale and impact on wellbeing at not being able to provide the best care possible.

6.5 PERSISTENCE OF AVOIDABLE HARM

There has been a growing recognition of the need to make significant improvements to patient safety developed in the 1980s and 1990s, and in the last 20 years, there have been a range of international and national initiatives aimed at reducing avoidable harm. Why then, despite the good work of many people over this time, has avoidable harm in health care, including that posed by HCAIs, remained a persistent, wide-scale problem? Avoidable harm in health care is, at its heart, a systemic issue. To make real progress in addressing this, it is necessary to tackle the following underlying system issues that allow it to persist.

6.6 SAFETY IS ONE PRIORITY OF MANY

Health and social care organisations have many strategic priorities. Often, patient safety is treated as one of these, weighed against others, with organisations and individuals then deciding which take precedence, patient safety becoming a matter of choice.

6.7 FEW SAFETY STANDARDS

Everyday practices in health care can be inconsistent, with no clear definition for what "good" looks like for patient safety. Organisations and regulators lack the means or commitment to set and manage consistent standards for patient safety performance.

6.8 NOT DESIGNING SAFE SYSTEMS

When designing and developing new healthcare procedures, processes, products and systems, too often patient safety considerations are an afterthought, rather than being a key element built into every step of the process.

6.9 BLAME CULTURE AND FEAR

Too often in health care we instead see organisational cultures which seek to assign blame when things go wrong, making patient harm more likely to happen again. It is widely acknowledged that to ensure patient safety issues are consistently reported and acted on, staff need to feel safe to do so and work in an organisational culture that supports and promotes this. Errors that lead to harm are invariably systems issues, and that personal accountability and blame will not address the underlying causes of avoidable harm.

6.10 PATIENTS NOT ENGAGED

Too often health care is designed and delivered around the traditional idea that the patient is the passive participant in the care process. This often results in patients having limited ability to participate in their care either because they are not informed about the stages of their treatment journey, what they should expect to happen, how to contribute to decision-making and how to escalate concerns in real time or if things go wrong. A recurring theme that emerges from investigations into serious patient safety incidents is that concerns raised by patients and family members are not acted on, and when harm occurs, they are left out of the investigation process.

6.11 LACK OF LEADERSHIP

Deficiencies in patient safety leadership, which undermine efforts to address avoidable harm, manifest themselves in a number of different ways. At a system level, in many countries around the world, there remains a lack of clarity about who is leading for patient safety, with organisations often operating within a fragmented and disconnected landscape. This can create difficulties in identifying and tackling patient safety issues, which require a system-wide response, even in some of the most advanced and well-resourced healthcare systems.

At an organisational level, we lack models for leadership and governance for patient safety that set clear standards and behaviours for our leaders. Simply put, there is no common view as to what it means to lead for patient safety. Patient safety is not always embedded into governance and risk management processes, and organisational leaders do not consistently model patient safety behaviours and promulgate these from the top down.

6.12 FAILURE TO LEARN AND ACT

Too often when effective solutions are found to prevent avoidable harm, there is simply a lack of means by which we share these more widely. This gap between learning and implementation means that while we may we know what improves patient safety, this information can often remain siloed in specific organisations and healthcare systems, resulting in patients continuing to experience harm from problems that have already been addressed by others (Patient Safety Learning 2022a).

REFLECTIVE EXERCISE

Before reading on, consider each of the seven underlying system issues that contribute to the persistence of avoidable harm. Which do you think are most relevant to the ongoing problem of HAIs? Do you work in an organisation that has a supportive culture for IPC? What would a culture that valued IPC look like? Is IPC embedded into governance and risk management structures?

6.13 THE NEED FOR A SYSTEMS APPROACH

How do we tackle the systemic causes of avoidable harm? In the report *A Blueprint for Action*, Patient Safety Learning set out the need for a transformation in the approach to patient safety, recognising this as a core purpose of health and social care (Patient Safety Learning 2019). Underpinned by systemic analysis and evidence, it identified six foundations of safe care for patients and practical actions to address them (Box 6.1).

BOX 6.1   THE SIX FOUNDATIONS OF SAFE CARE FOR PATIENTS

1. **Shared Learning**—organisations should set and deliver goals for learning, report on progress and share their insights widely for action.
2. **Leadership**—the importance of overarching leadership and governance for patient safety is emphasised.
3. **Professionalising Patient Safety**—organisations need to set and delivery high standards for patient safety. These need to be used by regulators to inform their assessment of whether organisations are doing enough to prevent avoidable harm and assess whether they are safe.
4. **Patient Engagement**—to ensure patients are valued and engaged in patient safety, at the point of care, if things go wrong and for redesigning health care for safety.
5. **Data and Insight**—better measurement and reporting of patient safety performance, both quantitative as well as qualitative
6. **Just Culture**—all organisations should publish goals and deliver programmes to eliminate blame and fear, introduce or deepen a just culture and measure and report progress.

6.14 CREATING SAFER SYSTEMS

In implementing these foundations of safe care, we also need to be aware of the practical complications that can come with improving patient safety in complex operating environments such as health care.

The hierarchy of improvement intervention effectiveness is a helpful model in this regard. On one end of the hierarchy are approaches that are systems based, such as forcing functions and automation. These can often be the most effective solutions but the hardest to implement as they require new ways of thinking and working, resources and organisational commitment. On the other end of the hierarchy are people-focused interventions, such as checklists, training and education, simpler to implement but less effective as they do not address the wider systems issues at hand (Toma et al. 2020).

It is also important to be aware of the difference between "Work-as-imagined" and "Work-as-done" and the implications of this for patient safety. "Work-as-imagined" describes what should happen under normal working conditions. "Work-as-done" describes what happens in practice, how work unfolds over time in complex contexts (Hollnagel 2017).

The gap between "Work-as-imagined" and "Work-as-done" is often where patient safety initiatives and products can come undone. In seeking to improve patient safety and reduce avoidable harm, it is vital to engage with how work takes place on the ground, and not solely rely on the idea of how it should take place.

6.15 SYSTEMS THINKING AND IPC

How does taking a systems-based approach to patient safety, making this a core purpose of health care, relate to IPC? Later, two examples are considered, one where systems thinking has been applied to an IPC issue, hand hygiene and another where it has not but could benefit from this, surgical site infections.

6.16 HAND HYGIENE

A small but crucial intervention, hand hygiene is a key measure in preventing HCAI and has had a particularly high prominence during the COVID-19 pandemic of 2020 (Storr 2021). Hand hygiene at the right moment can be a powerful intervention in stopping the spread of infection in health care settings. However, while a seemingly simple action on a personal level, as would be suggested by the hierarchy of improvement intervention effectiveness, looking at this as a primarily people-focused intervention limits its effective implementation. Hand hygiene is far from a new concept in IPC, and many healthcare organisations around the world have clearly established policies and guidelines in this respect. However, there are consistent difficulties in its implementation, and recent evidence highlights the ongoing challenge in achieving a culture in health care that supports hand hygiene improvement (de Kraker et al. 2022). The need for taking systems-level approaches to tackle this problem has been recognised in the development of the *WHO Multimodal Hand Hygiene Improvement Strategy*, aimed to assist organisations in implementing improvements to hand hygiene (WHO 2009). It emphasises the importance on not solely focusing on a people-centred approach but instead taking a wider system view:

> System change is a particularly important priority for healthcare facilities starting on their journey of hand hygiene improvement activities, assuming and expecting that the entire necessary infrastructure is put in place promptly. However, it is also essential that health-care facilities revisit the necessary infrastructure on a regular basis to ensure handwashing and hand hygiene facilities live up to a high standard on an ongoing basis.

The implementation of this broader approach, tackling hand hygiene as a system-level issue, has been shown to significantly improve compliance and knowledge of healthcare workers regarding hand hygiene (Allegranzi et al. 2013).

6.17 SURGICAL SITE INFECTIONS

A significant cause of HCAIs are surgical site infections (SSIs), occurring after surgery. As with hand hygiene, this is not a new IPC issue, with extensive guidance available on an international and national basis for healthcare professionals and organisations (WHO 2018a, Molnlycke 2020). There are various methods aimed at the prevention of infection in the operating theatre that have been shown to reduce the risk of such infections, such as avoiding shaving the operative site and appropriate use of preoperative antibiotics (WHO 2018b). WHO goes on to describe SSIs to be among the most preventable HCAIs but emphasise that they continue to represent a significant burden in terms of patient morbidity and mortality and additional costs to health systems and service payers worldwide. Reduction of SSI requires an understanding of human behaviours, and approaches should be grounded in social and implementation science theory supported by an appropriate infrastructure and environment, including a multimodal strategy described previously (Allegranzi et al. 2018).

6.18 SUPPORTING A SYSTEMS APPROACH TO PATIENT SAFETY AND IPC

Turning back towards the broader issues of developing a systems approach to patient safety and IPC, here we will focus on four key areas in more detail: shared learning, leadership and patient safety standards, culture, human factors and ergonomics.

6.19 SHARED LEARNING

If we are to move towards a systems-approach to patient safety and IPC, a key element required to achieve this will be ensuring that people and organisations share learning when they respond to incidents of avoidable harm and when they develop good practice for making care safer. One important aspect of this is enabling people and organisations to share learning and good practice. Patient Safety Learning created an online patient safety platform to support shared learning, *the hub* (Patient Safety Learning 2022b). Designed by and for patient safety professionals, clinicians and patients, the hub offers a powerful combination of tools, resources, stories, ideas, case studies and good practice to anyone who wants to make care safer for patients.

During the COVID-19 pandemic, the hub was used to share a range of new and developing patient safety and IPC resources, such as updated government guidance on IPC for seasonal respiratory infections in health and care settings and guidance to help facilitate visits to care and nursing homes. It is vital to develop and spread more ways to share IPC and patient safety learning and good practice if we are to overcome good practice being restricted to particular organisations or regions.

6.20 LEADERSHIP

In moving towards a systems approach to improving patient safety, the quality of the overarching leadership and governance is a key aspect of this. Good leadership can be a key driver of positive organisational culture in health care, but likewise, poor to absent leadership can have the opposite effect. There needs to be clarity on who leads for patient safety and common standards as to what is meant by this for providers, regulators, commissioners, and policymakers.

At a system level, there is a need for a model for leadership and governance for patient safety with clear roles and responsibilities. In an example of how such responsibilities might be rationalised in a complex and geographically dispersed healthcare system, in the United States there are new calls to create a federal independence agency, the National Patient Safety Board (National Patient Safety Board 2022). Modelled on similar bodies in other industries, there is a growing coalition of healthcare bodies now supporting this as a way to improve patient safety leadership at a system level.

At an organisational level, too often we see signs that on safety issues, boards and organisational leaders often wait to be told if they are safe or not by regulators rather than taking proactive steps. What is needed is for organisations to take ownership for safety—develop their own strategies based on their vision and ambition for change/achieving patient safety goals and informed by their own assessment of their baseline performance and a targeted and prioritised action plan. Then when regulators review, they are reflecting on this wider context and assessing against these plans, not just specific and operational key lines of enquiry.

6.21 PATIENT SAFETY STANDARDS

As mentioned earlier, one of the underlying causes of systemic harm is an inconsistency of everyday healthcare practices. This has been compounded by the historic lack of precision in defining what "good" looks like for patient safety and resulted in challenges in the development and application of standards for patient safety.

Patient Safety Learning is currently working on the development of organisational and system standards for patient safety in seeking to address this. This is based on the belief that by adopting and implementing comprehensive patient safety standards, organisations will be able to deliver safer care and embed a commitment to patient safety throughout their work. This would also enable patients, leaders, clinicians, the wider public and regulators to assess their progress and performance in improving patient safety. The aim is that these will help to deliver enhanced, evidence-based safety outcomes and behaviours.

6.22 CULTURE

Another area where it is vital to take a systems-approach to patient safety is culture. Organisational cultures that seek to assign blame when things go wrong make patient harm more likely to happen again. Blame culture incentivises people to cover up errors, rather than reporting them, and often singles out individuals rather than tackling the systemic causes of harm.

To improve patient safety, there is a need to move towards a Just Culture, a culture less focused on blame and one that considers the wider systemic issues that result in avoidable harm, enabling healthcare professionals to report issues without fear of retribution. This is an increasingly familiar concept in healthcare; however there is a significant difference between endorsing this approach in policy and implementing it in practice. To tackle avoidable harm, health systems and organisations need to proactively take steps to create an environment where individuals are supported in raising and resolving concerns, addressing incidents of unsafe care with empathy, respect and rigour. At a system level, national bodies need to enable the sharing of good practice and examples of where improvements have been made to create safer organisational cultures. They also need to be able to identify poorly performing organisations and intervene to make improvements. Organisations need to develop and publish goals to create and sustain a Just Culture, measuring and reporting on their progress in a transparent way. There also needs to be proactive efforts to ensure staff have the guidance, resources and support to speak up about safety issues.

6.23 HUMAN FACTORS AND ERGONOMICS

There are many cases where avoidable harm in health care is the result of systemic problems which have poor design at their core. Human Factors and ergonomics expertise are hugely important in understanding human performance in health and social care and can help to identify risks of avoidable harm and the solutions needed to ensure patient safety. Human Factors is defined by the International Ergonomics Association as:

> The scientific discipline concerned with the understanding of interactions among humans and other elements of a system, and the profession that applies theory, principles, data, and methods to design in order to optimize human well-being and overall system performance.
>
> International Ergonomics Association (2022)

Human factors and ergonomics approaches are already applied widely in other safety critical industries, such as energy, rail and aviation. By applying human factors to health care, the intention is to ensure that systems, products and services are designed to make them easier, safer and more effective for people to use. Embedding human factors as part of a systems-approach to tackling avoidable harm and improving patient safety might result in the following:

- Organisations have specialist patient safety and human factors experts in executive and non-executive roles on the board and leadership teams.
- Human factors and systems thinking inform the safe design, safety management and approaches to investigating unsafe care.
- Incident investigation and implementation of improvement strategies being led by people who have undertaken recognised, accredited training, which includes systems and human factors expertise.

For more on the relevance and application of human factors to IPC, refer to Chapter 10.

6.24 CONCLUSION

Preventing avoidable harm in health care remains a key global health challenge, described by the G20 Health and Development Partnership as the "Overlooked Pandemic." This chapter has set out that at the root of this issue lies a range of underlying systemic issues in current approaches to patient safety, which need to be addressed with a systems-approach if health care is to be made safer. To achieve this requires a fundamental transformation in how patient safety is approached, with patient safety being treated as core to the purpose of health and social care. This broader change will provide a context in which patient safety and IPC programmes and interventions can be developed and good practice widely shared and implemented to ensure patients receive effective and safe care.

6.25 REFERENCES

Allegranzi, B. et al. (2013). Global implementation of WHO's multimodal strategy for improvement of hand hygiene: A quasi-experimental study. *The Lancet: Infectious Diseases*, 1 October, *13*(10). www.thelancet.com/journals/laninf/article/PIIS1473-3099(13)70163-4/fulltext

Allegranzi, B., Aiken, A. M., Zeynep Kubilay, N., Nthumba, P., Barasa, J., Okumu, G., Mugarura, R., Elobu, A., Jombwe, J., Maimbo, M., Musowoya, J., Gayet-Ageron, A., & Berenholtz, S. M. (2018). A multimodal infection control and patient safety intervention to reduce surgical site infections in Africa: A multicentre, before-after, cohort study. *The Lancet. Infectious Diseases*, *18*(5), 507–515. https://doi.org/10.1016/S1473-3099(18)30107-5

Andel, C., Davidow, S. L., Hollander, M., & Moreno, D. A. (2012). The economics of health care quality and medical errors. *Journal of Health Care Finance*, *39*(1), 39–50.

de Kraker, M. E. A., Tartari, E., Tomczyk, S., Twyman, A., Francioli, L. C., Cassini, A., Allegranzi, B., & Pittet, D. (2022). Implementation of hand hygiene in health-care facilities: Results from the WHO hand hygiene self-assessment framework global survey 2019. *Lancet Infectious Diseases*. Published Online February 21, 2022. https://doi.org/10.1016/S1473-3099(21)00618-6

G20 (2021). The G20 health and development partnership, the overlooked pandemic: How to transform patent safety and save healthcare systems, 18 March. www.ssdhub.org/the-overlooked-pandemic/

Gonzales, K. (2010). Medication administration errors and the pediatric population: A systematic search of the literature. *Journal of Pediatric Nursing*, *25*(6), 555–565. https://doi.org/10.1016/j.pedn.2010.04.002

Hollnagel, E. (2017). Can we ever imagine how work is done? *Hindsight*, 25 Summer. www.eurocontrol.int/sites/default/files/publication/files/hindsight25.pdf

International Ergonomics Association (2022). What is ergonomics? Last Accessed 4 March 2022. https://iea.cc/what-is-ergonomics/

Molnlycke (2020). Time to act: A state of the nation report on surgical site infections in the UK, December. www.pslhub.org/learn/patient-safety-in-health-and-care/high-risk-areas/surgery/surgical-site-infections/time-to-act-a-state-of-the-nation-report-on-surgical-site-infections-in-the-uk-december-2020-r3895/

National Patient Safety Board (2022). About. Last Accessed 1 March 2022. https://npsb.org/about/

OECD & SPSC (2020). The economics of patient safety, October. www.oecd.org/health/health-systems/Economics-of-Patient-Safety-October-2020.pdf

Patient Safety Learning (2019). The patient-safe future: A blueprint for action. Report. https://s3-eu-west-1.amazonaws.com/ddme-psl/content/A-Blueprint-for-Action-240619.pdf?mtime=20190701143409

Patient Safety Learning (2022a). Mind the implementation gap: The persistence of avoidable harm in the NHS, 7 April. https://s3-eu-west-1.amazonaws.com/ddme-psl/Mindtheimplementationgap_ThepersistenceofavoidableharmintheNHS_2022-04–07–121554_vhao.pdf

Patient Safety Learning (2022b). The hub. Last Accessed 1 March 2022.

Storr, J. (2021). Seconds save lives—let's not forget that: A blog by Julie Storr, 5 May. www.pslhub.org/learn/improving-patient-safety/seconds-save-lives-%E2%80%93-let%E2%80%99s-not-forget-that-a-blog-by-julie-storr-r4532/

Toma, M., Blamey, A., Mahal, D., Gray, N. M., Allison, L., Thakore, S., & Bowie, P. (2020). Multi-method evaluation of a national clinical fellowship programme to build leadership capacity for quality improvement. *BMJ Open Quality*, *9*(4), e000978. https://doi.org/10.1136/bmjoq-2020-000978

WHO (2009). A guide to the implementation of the WHO multimodal hand hygiene improvement strategy, 9 February. www.who.int/publications/i/item/a-guide-to-the-implementation-of-the-who-multimodal-hand-hygiene-improvement-strategy

WHO (2016a). *Guidelines on core components of infection prevention and control programmes at the national and acute health care facility level*. Geneva: World Health Organization.

WHO (2016b). *Healthcare without avoidable infections: The critical role of infection prevention and control*. Geneva: World Health Organization.

WHO (2018a). *Implementation manual to support the prevention of surgical site infections at the facility level—turning recommendations into practice (interim version)*. Geneva: World Health Organization (WHO/HIS/SDS/2018.18).

WHO (2018b). *Global guidelines for the prevention of surgical site infection*, 2nd edition. Geneva: World Health Organization.

WHO (2019). Patient safety fact file, September. www.who.int/features/factfiles/patient_safety/patient-safety-fact-file.pdf?ua=1

WHO (2021). Global patient safety action plan 2021–2030, 3 August. www.who.int/publications/i/item/9789240032705

Communicating With Compassion—Service User Perspectives

7

Melissa Kleine-Bingham,
Nana Afriyie Mensah Abrampah,
Louis Ako-Egbe and Shamsuzzoha Babar Syed

Contents

7.1 WHAT IS COMPASSIONATE CARE?

While many would agree that compassion should be considered as part of the provision and the experience of care, it is not always well understood. Increasingly, there is growing agreement that compassion can be defined as the emotional response to another's pain or suffering, followed by a desire to take action to alleviate that suffering (Berlant 2004). Empathy, which is the "ability to understand and share the feelings of another" (The New Oxford English Dictionary 2001), detects and mirrors emotions and experiences and is the precursor to compassion.

As such, compassion is often seen as the ability to empathise but also requires action to alleviate suffering, which differentiates it as a step beyond empathy. Box 7.1 considers compassion within the context of health worker competencies.

DOI: 10.1201/9781003379393-9

BOX 7.1

"Ethical, respectful and *compassionate care*, and the fundamentals of systems thinking, and quality improvement should be additional core competencies" [for health professionals].

Kruck et al. 2018

7.2 THE POSITIVE IMPACT OF COMPASSION ON HEALTH AND WELLBEING

Only compassionate care recognizes the need for quality health services in marginalized communities or conflict areas.

(Ministry of Health, Quality Directorate)

Recent research by Roberts et al. (2019) provides an increased understanding on the direct effects of compassionate care on health service delivery (provision of care) and client perception (experience of care). For example, when patients perceive their healthcare provider as being compassionate, health outcomes improve (Trzeciak & Mazzarelli 2019; WHO 2018a). This has been illustrated by several studies which show that compassionate care can reduce ailments such as migraines (Attar & Chandramani 2012) while also enhancing immune response (Rakel et al. 2009), improve patient compliance with prescriptive therapies (Kim et al. 2004) and reduce depression and improve the quality of one's life (Burns & Nolen-Hoeksema 1992; Neumann et al. 2007; Zachariae et al. 2003). Conversely, a lack of compassion has been shown to increase health spending and resource utilization (Schulz et al. 2007; Sinclair et al. 2016; Papadopoulos et al. 2017), while compassion fatigue (or "burnout") among health providers can greatly reduce quality of care (Hamilton et al. 2016).

Further, compassionate care has the potential to break down barriers to healthcare access. This is particularly poignant in relation to an individual's willingness to seek health services within a multicultural environment. Some suggest that when a healthcare professional is seeing a patient from a different cultural background or religion, compassion is the main element that drives them to treat the patient with the highest quality of care that they can provide (WHO 2019). Thus, compassion can be used to develop common understanding within a multicultural environment.

7.3 THE LANGUAGE OF COMPASSION

Careful consideration must also be given to the linguistic nuances around the word *compassion*. A scoping review of compassion terminology used across the health sector and within varied settings revealed the complexity associated with the term (WHO 2018a). For example, the Spanish translation of the word "compassion" links to pity and hierarchical treatment, which patients do not want from their healthcare providers. In this context, the word "empathy" is preferred. This brings to light why interpretation of the terms used and definitional concepts behind these terms are such a critical area of enquiry.

Compassionate care is based on values and ethics of serving patients and can further influence health, healing and patient satisfaction by respecting rights and choices of patients through supportive communication, actions and attitudes. Compassion as a code of ethics includes such rights as conveying the patient plan of care, patient's having decision-making authority within their plan of care and lastly to choose the course of treatment (Berhe et al. 2017).

7.4 COMPASSION AND QUALITY OF CARE

Compassion is central to and underpins action on delivering quality health services. Quality health services diagrammed in Figure 7.1 are fundamental to achieving universal health coverage (UHC) and meeting the sustainable development goals (SDGs). Quality health services should be effective, safe and people-centred (WHO 2018b). Additionally, in order to realise the benefits of quality health care, health services must also be timely, equitable, integrated and efficient. The 2018 report by WHO, the Organization for Economic Co-operation and Development (OECD) and the World Bank, titled *Delivering quality health services: a global imperative for universal health coverage* (WHO 2018b), clearly articulates that care must be effective and safe, while keeping to the preferences

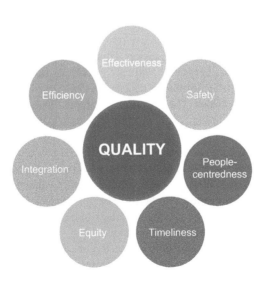

FIGURE 7.1 Key domains for quality of care

and needs of the people and communities being served. By involving people and communities in their own plan of care, health outcomes improve, and people suffer fewer complications and enjoy better health and wellbeing. It is within this context that the role of compassion can be considered.

Each of the three key domains involved in quality of health services—effectiveness, safety and people-centredness—have clear linkages to compassionate care. Providing quality health services to everyone, every time, requires that the care provided be evidence-based, for it to be *effective*. Effective treatment includes applying appropriate interventions when delivering care with compassion and learning from current and past experiences and feeding perspectives from individuals into the development of evidence-based guidelines. Everyone's needs and unique circumstances require attention in order to avoid harm to the patient. For health care to be *safe* requires health care professionals giving special attention to a patient's medical history and clinical experiences—compassion can enhance the desire for and action towards safety in diverse areas, for example, safe surgical care or medication administration. People-centred care consciously adopts the individual's perspective and needs as well as that of the families and communities as a participant in trusted health systems; this requires that individuals have the knowledge and support they need to make decisions and actively participate in their own care with compassion embedded within its fabric (WHO 2016). Compassionate care, which involves placing the person before the disease or illness, is truly vital in this drive for quality of care.

Globally, increasing attention has been drawn to the *lack* of compassionate care in healthcare settings. In particular, the 2013 Francis Inquiry report of the Mid Staffordshire NHS Foundation Trust in the UK generated intense scrutiny of how compassionate practices are conducted in healthcare facilities, the barriers to compassionate care and why compassion is so central to patient experience and quality. Conversation on compassion has since been intensified, seeking to universalize its definition, capture patient and provider experiences with compassionate care, understand barriers to compassionate care and create effective, science-based interventions for cultivating compassionate care.

Compassion has a critical role to play in advancing health systems to deliver quality health care, improve performance and achieve universal health coverage. Indeed, the concept of universality is imbued with compassion. This focus on compassion when combined with how engagement occurs between healthcare providers, service users, their families and communities affect trust, information sharing, decision-making and directly impacts on the quality of health services. The absence of compassion can cause clinical errors, high rates of health worker absenteeism and burnout, poor patient experience, physician disengagement and attrition. Compassionate care also has the potential to inform national authorities on how to advance on improving the quality of care at all levels of the health system through the engagement of healthcare providers, service users, their families and communities in the design, delivery, implementation and evaluation of health services. Such an approach can enhance the trust placed in health services. A focus on compassionate health services, allows people's needs and values to be placed at the forefront of care, thus improving the overall quality of health services.

There is a well-acknowledged emphasis on the need for those who provide health care to understand the patient's physical, sociological and psychological health needs and the social, cultural and historical factors that have shaped them (WHO 2016). This allows the provider to recognise and value the patient's preferences and beliefs and reorganize health services to better support them across the health continuum and life course. People-centred approaches to service delivery design place emphasis on the person across all health service delivery efforts, regardless of where care is delivered. The ethos of a person-centred approach is captured as a key theme surrounding the renewed global focus on primary health care (WHO 2020): meeting people's health needs throughout their lives, addressing the broader determinants of health through multisectoral policy and action and empowering individuals, families and communities to take charge of their own health (WHO 2021). This is done with the recognition that throughout the course of a person's life, primary care can meet 80–90% of one's health needs (WHO 2018c). A focus on compassion can support the necessary transformation required to focus on high quality primary health care for everyone, everywhere.

7.5 COMPASSIONATE LEADERSHIP AND THE HEALTH SYSTEM

Engagement of leadership across all levels of the health system is a key feature to institutionalize a culture of quality across the health system. Leadership is also fundamental in progressing a compassionate environment and, moreover, compassionate care. Compassionate leadership has enormous benefits to an organisation by improving creativity, workers' productivity and retention and reducing burnouts, for example (de Zulueta 2015). When leadership supports a compassionate environment, those working within the environment have opportunities for relational development both as a team and individually (Bridges & Fuller 2015). Bridges & Fuller go on to state that leaders have profound impact on optimising and sustaining team capacity to develop and support compassionate interactions among staff. In recent years, compassionate training programmes are becoming globally available. One such leadership programme, "Creating Learning Environments for Compassionate Care," is a four-month practice development programme for professionals and service users in health and social care settings in the UK. Within this programme, there is emphasis on developing and embedding sustainable management, leadership and team relational practices in areas such as dialogue, reflective learning and mutual support.

Further, strong leadership supporting a compassionate environment can mitigate many of the challenges and barriers to fostering a compassionate working space. Such challenges may be inadequate staffing; dysfunctional incentive structures relating to performance targets unrelated to compassion; lack of values, strategic priorities and leadership style at the top of organizations (Mannion 2014). Mannion also concludes that in health facilities, there can be additional barriers such as shorter lengths of stay for patients combined with changing shift patterns of staff. Leadership and management at all levels of the health system can influence and provide strategic direction in order to overcome many of these barriers.

Compassionate leadership involves a revealing of self (including vulnerability) as this build's courage, trust, skills and values within the organisation and consequently enhances self-compassion and mindfulness. Some of the solutions identified to support compassionate care included putting strong leadership in place, encouraging positive role modelling for junior staff and trainees and continued education to support therapeutic communication skills (WHO 2019). As such, there is clear need for compassionate leaders at all levels of the health systems (health facility, district/subnational and national) as well as at the global level (Germer & Neff 2013).

At the facility level, compassion can be placed as a compass for delivering quality at the point of care. Further, compassion provides an important basis for leading worker-to-worker interactions that stimulate a culture of quality. Subnational authorities have a role to play in delivering compassionate care to communities and clients/patients of health services, ensuring that the organisation of quality health services is conducted based on principles of compassion. National leadership can benefit from embedding compassion within national policies and legislation with clear guidance on how to operationalize these at the subnational level.

At the global level, the inclusion of compassion as part of normative documents and technical guidance provided to national-level leadership, and across implementation cycles can serve to scale-up the benefits of compassion. Further, the global level plays a key role in shaping the learning agenda, ensuring that innovative approaches on compassion are identified and shared.

Competency development on compassion is a cross-cutting function across all levels, ensuring that the health system is developing and sustaining a compassionate health workforce (Figure 7.2).

The interrelationship between each level of the health system is presented from the perspective of a clinician in the country case study (Box 7.2 words of compassion at the frontlines).

In summary, leaders should strive towards creating systems that can mitigate workplace anxiety, support for the individuals involved and model positive adaptive responses to challenges (de Zulueta 2015). The scoping and codevelopment report on compassion from the WHO Global Learning Laboratory highlights that this can be achieved by governments, organisations and communities through shifting workplace paradigms to include models of leadership that embraces workplace cultural diversity and views the organisation as a complex living system and leadership as adaptive, shared and distributed

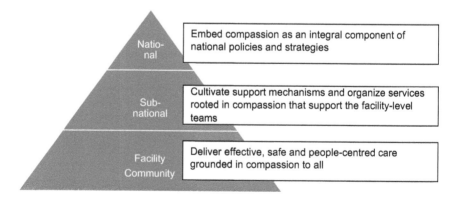

FIGURE 7.2 Compassion across the levels

(de Zulueta 2015; WHO 2019). While leadership is instrumental in facilitating a compassionate environment, it is not always easy to exemplify. Some of the challenges for leaders to be compassionate are the "desire to save the world, lack of boundaries, lack of self-compassion and burnouts" (Addiss 2018). Additionally, many leaders fear to appear vulnerable as this exposes their emotions and denotes uncertainty and risk. This can, however, be turned into a strength for future-focused compassionate leaders.

BOX 7.2   COUNTRY CASE STUDY: WORDS OF COMPASSION AT THE FRONTLINES

The healthcare delivery environment in Cameroon, like many in resource-limited settings, is very challenging. Poor health infrastructure, inadequate skilled and motivated personnel and worsening sociopolitical climate are some of the challenges impairing the delivery of quality health care.

As a medical practitioner and district health manager in a remote district in Cameroon, it was challenging to be compassionate to colleagues and patients in a system which was void of compassion for the workforce. However, we decided to create a safe haven for ourselves by cultivating compassion within the district team (which is charged with supervising and building capacity for health facility personnel, including managers) and by extension to the patients. We adopted diverse approaches, for example establishing social platforms—regular meetings, social media platforms—for personnel to share events in their personal lives (bereavements, anniversaries and birth celebrations) beyond usual office/health facility work. Through these platforms, we could support and share in the mourning and happiness of colleagues financially, physically and morally. The district created a solidarity fund to support staff in times of financial crisis. All these innovations helped strengthen the compassionate bond between district staff and health facility teams, created a unique environment for work and reignited trust within the team. Staff confidence was renewed, and untapped skills were reawakened.

By building this microcosm of compassion, the district experienced an improvement in its performance regarding the timeliness and accuracy of reporting. Health facility managers in hard-to-reach communities devised new ways to ensure that their monthly reports were received at the district health service before deadlines. We received few reports of staff burnouts or abandonment of posts of work.

As a clinician, a key attribute of compassion which made a difference in my practice was the ability to listen to my patients effectively (uninterrupted attention). They felt heard, loved and left my office satisfied, even if my clinical intervention was minimal.

This demonstrates that as individuals (patients or providers of health care), we all yearn for compassion. We need to feel heard and loved. We need health systems that have living consciences, able to palpate, diagnose and respond to our needs first as HUMANS, then as health workers with whitecoats and stethoscopes.

7.6 REFLECTIVE EXERCISE—EVERYDAY COMPASSION

Chapter 8 builds on the foundations established here and starts to consider some of these principles and concepts in relation to real-world IPC situations. Before moving on, consider the following questions that have been triggered by the content of this chapter:

1. Policies and guidelines—do IPC policies and guidelines in the place you work make explicit reference to compassion?
2. Opportunities to learn more about compassion and health care—is compassion addressed within any training or education sessions you have attended recently, in any discipline?
3. If you had to describe a compassionate leader—what traits do you think they would possess?
4. Can you remember a recent situation where yourself or a colleague demonstrated compassion in a healthcare context—what actions or words made this memorable?
5. How do you think health workers can be supported to be compassionate? For example, is compassion part of your core competencies? What do you see as the pros and cons of positioning compassion within health worker competencies?

7.7 REFERENCES

Addiss, D. G. (2018). Spiritual themes and challenges in global health. *The Journal of Medical Humanities*, 39(3), 337–348.

Attar, H. S., & Chandramani, S. (2012). Impact of physician empathy on migraine disability and migraineur compliance. *Annals of Indian Academy of Neurology*, 15(Suppl 1), S89–S94.

Berhe, H., Berhe, H., Bayray, A., Gigar, G., Godifay, H., & Gebretekle, G. B. (2017). Status of caring, respectful and compassionate health care practice in Tigtai regional state: Patients' perspective. *International Journal of Caring Science*, September–December, 10(3), 1119.

Berlant, L. (2004). Compassion (and withholding). In L. Berlant (ed.), *Compassion—The Culture and Politics of an Emotion*, 1st edition. Oxon: Routledge Publishing, 1–13.

Bridges, J., & Fuller, A. (2015). Creating learning environments for compassionate care: A programme to promote compassionate care by health and social care teams. *International Journal of Older People Nursing*, 10(1), 48–58.

Burns, D. D., & Nolen-Hoeksema, S. (1992). Therapeutic empathy and recovery from depression in cognitive-behavioral therapy: A structural equation model. *Journal of Consulting and Clinical Psychology*, 60(3), 441–449.

de Zulueta, P. C. (2015). Developing compassionate leadership in health care: An integrative review. *Journal of Healthcare Leadership*, 8, 1–10.

Germer, C. K., & Neff, K. D. (2013). Self-compassion in clinical practice. *Journal of Clinical Psychology*, 69(8), 856–867.

Hamilton, S., Tran, V., & Jamieson, J. (2016). Compassion fatigue in emergency medicine: The cost of caring. *Emergency Medicine Australasia: EMA*, 28(1), 100–103.

Kim, S. S., Kaplowitz, S., & Johnston, M. V. (2004). The effects of physician empathy on patient satisfaction and compliance. *Evaluation & the Health Professions*, 27(3), 237–251.

Kruk, M. E., Gage, A. D., Arsenault, C., Jordan, K., Leslie, H. H., Roder-DeWan, S., Adeyi, O., Barker, P., Daelmans, B., Doubova, S. V., English, M., García-Elorrio, E., Guanais, F., Gureje, O., Hirschhorn, L. R., Jiang, L., Kelley, E., Lemango, E. T., Liljestrand, J., Malata, A., . . . Pate, M. (2018). High-quality health systems in the Sustainable development goals era: Time for a revolution. *The Lancet. Global Health*, 6(11), e1196–e1252. https://doi.org/10.1016/S2214-109X(18)30386-3

Mannion, R. (2014). Enabling compassionate healthcare: Perils, prospects and perspectives. *International Journal of Health Policy and Management*, 2(3), 115–117.

Neumann, M., Wirtz, M., Bollschweiler, E., Mercer, S. W., Warm, M., Wolf, J., & Pfaff, H. (2007). Determinants and patient-reported long-term outcomes of physician empathy in oncology: A structural equation modelling approach. *Patient Education and Counseling*, 69(1–3), 63–75.

The New Oxford English Dictionary (2001). Oxford: Oxford University Press.

Papadopoulos, I., Taylor, G., Ali, S., Aagard, M., Akman, O., Alpers, L. M., Apostolara, P., Biglete-Pangilinan, S., Biles, J., García, Á. M., González-Gil, T., Koulouglioti, C., Kouta, C., Krepinska, R., Kumar, B. N., Lesińska-Sawicka, M., Diaz, A., Malliarou, M., Nagórska, M., Nassim, S., . . . Zorba, A. (2017). Exploring nurses' meaning and experiences of compassion: An international online survey involving 15 countries. *Journal of Transcultural Nursing: Official Journal of the Transcultural Nursing Society*, 28(3), 286–295.

Rakel, D. P., Hoeft, T. J., Barrett, B. P., Chewning, B. A., Craig, B. M., & Niu, M. (2009). Practitioner empathy and the duration of the common cold. *Family Medicine*, 41(7), 494–501.

Roberts, B. W., Roberts, M. B., Yao, J., Bosire, J., Mazzarelli, A., & Trzeciak, S. (2019). Development and validation of a tool to measure patient assessment of clinical compassion. *JAMA Network Open*, 2(5), e193976.

Schulz, R., Hebert, R. S., Dew, M. A., Brown, S. L., Scheier, M. F., Beach, S. R., Czaja, S. J., Martire, L. M., Coon, D., Langa, K. M., Gitlin, L. N., Stevens, A. B., & Nichols, L. (2007). Patient suffering and caregiver compassion: New opportunities for research, practice, and policy. *The Gerontologist*, 47(1), 4–13.

Sinclair, S., Norris, J. M., McConnell, S. J., Chochinov, H. M., Hack, T. F., Hagen, N. A., McClement, S., & Bouchal, S. R. (2016). Compassion: A scoping review of the healthcare literature. *BMC Palliative Care*, 15, 6.

Trzeciak, S., & Mazzarelli, A. (2019). *Compassionomics—The Revolutionary Scientific Evidence that Caring Makes a Difference*. Pensacola, FL: The Studer Group, LLC.

WHO (2016). *World Health Organization. Framework on Integrated, People-Centered Health Services*. 15 April. Available at: https://apps.who.int/gb/ebwha/pdf_files/WHA69/A69_39-en.pdf

WHO (2018a). *Scoping Report: Compassion and Quality of Care. World Health Organization*. Geneva: WHO. Available at: https://worldhealthorg.sharepoint.com/sites/ws-GLL4QUHC/compassion/SitePages/Consultation.aspx

WHO (2018b). *Delivering Quality Health Services: A Global Imperative for Universal Health Coverage*. World Health Organization, Organisation for Economic Co-operation and Development, the World Bank. Geneva: World Health Organization. Available at: http://apps.who.int/iris/bitstream/handle/10665/272465/9789241513906-eng.pdf?ua=1

WHO (2018c). *World Health Organization. 2018 Primary Health Care Conference*. Available at: www.who.int/docs/default-source/primary-health-care-conference/quality.pdf

WHO (2019). *Compassion—The Health of Quality Health Services: Scoping and Co-development Report*. World Health Organization—The WHO Global Learning Laboratory for Quality UHC. Geneva: WHO. Available at: https://worldhealthorg.sharepoint.com/sites/ws-GLL4QUHC/compassion/SitePages/Consultation.aspx

WHO (2020). *World Health Organization, UNICEF. 2020. A Vision for Primary Health care in the 21st Century*. Available at: www.who.int/docs/default-source/primary-health/vision.pdf?sfvrsn=c3119034_2

WHO (2021). *World Health Organization. 2021. Primary Health Care Fact Sheet.* Available at: www.who.int/news-room/fact-sheets/detail/primary-health-care

Zachariae, R., Pedersen, C. G., Jensen, A. B., Ehrnrooth, E., Rossen, P. B., & von der Maase, H. (2003). Association of perceived physician communication style with patient satisfaction, distress, cancer-related self-efficacy, and perceived control over the disease. *British Journal of Cancer*, 88(5), 658–665.

The Weaponising of IPC and Its Heartbreaking Consequences

8

Julie Storr, Claire Kilpatrick and Sheila Hall

Contents

We protected them to death.

—Denise Gracely, Pennsylvania 2020
(Rubinkam 2021)

8.1 INTRODUCTION TO THE ISSUE

History is replete with examples of the inhumane treatment of people by people, and sometimes this happens in health care, sometimes in the midst of infectious disease outbreaks. The 1980s are remembered for the dark days of stigma against those with HIV and AIDS, and more recently similar patterns of stigmatisation have been reported in relation to other microorganisms in health care, meticillin-resistant *Staphylococcus aureus* (MRSA) and Ebola virus disease to name but two, with fear of contagion a key influencer of the stigmatisation.

In recent years, the need to consider compassion as a component of quality health services has come to the fore. Chapter 7 provides an outline of the case for compassion and its importance in the delivery and user experience of health care and should be read in conjunction with this chapter. The focus of what follows is on the COVID-19 pandemic and an examination and critique of the use of IPC to justify practices that at times lacked compassion. It therefore touches on compassion, quality and IPC, the latter being an important part of quality health care. The issues raised however also touch on matters of ageism, social justice, equity, ethics, humanity (including inhumanity) and mental health. Most of all, however, this chapter is concerned with the consequences of what people do in the name of IPC. The things that health workers do to prevent and control infection, the advice provided, the guidelines that outline the evidence-based best practices, how they are interpreted and implemented—rightly or wrongly—has consequences.

8.2 THE EMERGING COMPASSION AGENDA

A good starting point when focusing on compassion and health care can be found in the United Kingdom (UK) National Health Service (NHS). A major scandal centred around poor quality care and the associated avoidable death of patients in the 2000s resulted in an investigation and report, the findings of which brought to prominence issues around the lack of compassion and its consequences (Francis 2013; Martin & Dixon Woods 2014). A national, nurse-led strategy and initiative was born around that time that spoke about the importance of the "6Cs": care, courage, communication, competence, commitment and compassion (Department of Health 2012). In the United States of America (US), the need for compassion in health care was pioneered by the Schwartz Centre for Compassionate health care with their philosophy that the "smallest acts of kindness" by health workers can make "the unbearable bearable" for patients (Cornwell 2014). Compassion is not solely relevant to patient care. In an evaluation of the implementation of the 6Cs strategy, participants stated that compassion for patients is only sustainable where there is compassion for staff (O'Driscoll et al. 2018).

Recently, an interesting book, *Compassionomics* by Treciak and Mazarelli (2019), has taken the debate about the role of compassion in health care to a new level. These authors forensically dissect compassion and explore its utility in health care from the point of view of proving its evidence base and its impact on outcome. *Compassionomics* can be a helpful starting point since it begins by drilling in to what compassion is. The authors explain that most scientists define compassion as "the emotional response to another's pain or suffering, involving an authentic desire to help." But importantly they point out that it is different from empathy—empathy is the feeling and understanding part; what makes compassion different is that it involves action—taking action to address those feelings. Feeling empathy is a necessary precursor or prerequisite to motivate the action of compassion. Different areas of the brain are involved in both empathy and compassion. The authors suggest that compassion—responding to another's suffering—is the essence of what makes us human—if one lacks compassion, one is essentially lacking humanity.

8.3 A SLIPPERY SLOPE

Some decisions made in the name of IPC when subject to closer scrutiny are in fact based on a misunderstanding of IPC. IPC is sometimes used as a rationale to justify or legitimise edicts that in fact are not matters of IPC. In my previous book, a chapter titled "Just Infection Prevention and Control" (Storr 2016) aimed to spark a conversation on the rationale for a number of the things that are done in the name of IPC. In it I talked about the need to revise IPC strategies so that they are focused both on halting microbial transmission and harm to people, because that is the essence of IPC, but also that they do so from a holistic, rights- based perspective that takes account of dignity, of ethics, of humanity and of justice. The reader may have encountered the following, either as a recipient or an implementer: stopping the wearing of ties, a fixation on the length of a health workers' sleeve, banning visitors from sitting on patients' beds and even forbidding flowers and Christmas decorations—all in the name of following IPC rules. There is no hard evidence from an IPC perspective for any of these "rules," and while the impact of the bans or edicts is variable, some do have an effect on people's psychosocial wellbeing when in hospital, an illustration of the negative consequences not of microbes but of the prevention and control mechanisms employed in the name of IPC.

Moving up a gear, during the COVID-19 pandemic, IPC was used as a rationale to support a number of "preventative" measures that were promoted widely across health and social care in many countries. Focusing on settings beyond the acute hospital, as the pandemic took hold across the globe, care homes/long-term care facilities (LTCFs) imposed policies that excluded all families, often referred to as "visitors"—with no exceptions. In many cases this persisted for months, and for some, the months turned into years. In some cases, fuelled by IPC as the chief rationale, husbands and wives, parents and their children never saw each other again.

8.4 SPOTLIGHT ON THE CONSEQUENCE OF RESTRICTIONS TO CARE HOMES IN A PANDEMIC—A PERSONAL ACCOUNT

My interest was piqued on seeing some shocking reports on social media concerning these ongoing restriction of "visitors" to health and social care facilities. My response was to bring together a group of IPC experts and concerned individuals to issue an open letter that was published in the UK nursing press (Storr et al. 2020). The aim was to highlight the issue and start to present the case that IPC should enable, not prevent, safe interactions. This was followed by a similar letter in the *American Journal of Infection Control* (Storr et al. 2021) and later an opinion piece in the *BMJ* (Suárez-González & Storr 2021). The aim of these pieces was to bring attention to this evolving issue and in particular on the need for IPC experts in all countries to come together and try to rebalance the narrative so that a rightful emphasis on the technical, practical measures that need to be in place (i.e. the guidance) to keep people safe was not at the expense of a compassionate milieu.

What happened at this time was essentially about how IPC logic and guidance was interpreted (or misinterpreted), applied (or misapplied) and implemented (or erroneously implemented). The guidance itself was in many instances not at fault, and there are many causative factors at play that will be considered later. The open letter listed five considerations to help stimulate action on this:

1. The "rules" of IPC don't and shouldn't stop family members and close friends of residents entering LTCFs, even during periods of lockdown.
2. IPC should be used as an enabler and supporter of safe entry to LTCFs. The logic for this centred on the fact that all the precautionary measures being employed by workers in LTCFs could be applied by all others who needed entry in order to protect vulnerable residents.
3. Routinization and de-implementation presented a serious concern. The use of outdoor heaters to support outdoor "visits" by families in winter and the use of video call technology was becoming an unacceptable "norm." This is not the answer, and other more humane solutions are available.
4. IPC and compassionate care are not mutually exclusive, and there is an evidence-based case for lifting restrictions and bans and not just for immediate end-of-life situations.
5. Families provide (unpaid) care in many situations, and all IPC recommendations for paid caregivers can be applied. In summary, IPC should be applied as a force for good.

For the purposes of clarity, de-implementation can be defined as reducing or stopping the use of a health service or practice provided to patients by healthcare practitioners and systems and usually addresses ineffective, unproven, harmful, overused, inappropriate, and/or low-value health services and practices to mitigate patient harm and improve processes of care (Norton et al. 2017). The letter presented six actions targeted at nursing, care and residential home managers (LTCF managers), governments/local authorities, the IPC community, healthcare leaders, families and campaigning groups, to help progress a solution to the problem. Although mainly focused on the UK, signatories came from beyond the UK; however all were writing mainly from a high-income country perspective. I was subsequently contacted by colleagues in other countries, suggesting that similar challenges were faced beyond high-income contexts. The intention of these pieces was to empower and support those who were already lobbying for change—many of these were civil society groups that had started campaigning as a result of their own personal experiences. I was contacted by scores of individuals who shared with me their personal stories. One of those is summarised in Box 8.1.

**BOX 8.1   HOW WAS THE PANDEMIC ALLOWED TO CONCEAL
COMPASSION? A FEAR FOG THAT COVERED CRITICAL THINKING**

A reflection on my grandmother, Dora. A lady not shy from work over the years and enjoying alongside her husband a typical farming family life. A lady who had 5 children, 11 grandchildren and 20 great-grandchildren. Always food on the table whatever time of day you decided to arrive and the smell of a cake baking for visitors to enjoy with their cup of tea. Never a day went by without at least a couple of visitors. Involved in village life and loved chatting to her neighbours and attending the local community hall.

In early 2020 my grandmother was in the hospital. She had become frail, and mobility was declining. It was heartbreaking, but the decision was made that it was time for her to be cared for in a local nursing home. She accepted this and was reassured when told she could bring some of her items from home and that visitors would be able to come and go as often as she would like.

She transferred to the NH. All was going to plan until the news of the pandemic. What did this mean for the whole family unit? I reassured the family, saying with good IPC measures there should be no reason why visiting would be restricted. Suddenly it became apparent that visiting would be stopped. This was the most traumatic news to deliver to her and family members. She went from 95 years of family life to being cut off from everyone basically overnight. She questioned at one point, saying, "The government would never allow this to happen," and asked if the family were deserting her. She said she felt as if she was trapped in a prison situation. So many heartbroken family members and nothing that could be done. The helplessness was dreadful to witness.

Eight weeks went by with her seeing no family at all, and just a couple of days before she died it was agreed that her children could see her one last time. Did she know they were there? Did she forgive them for not visiting? Sadly, she died alone. Only ten people were allowed to attend her funeral. Her children and their partners attended an outdoor service, and her own sister had to stay away. Families have been robbed of precious times and left to deal with the trauma for the rest of their lives.

Jacq Cross, former infection prevention and control nurse

8.5 PROPORTIONALITY

A 2015 publication by the Global Network of WHO Collaborating Centres for Bioethics (WHO 2015) looked at restrictions on movement and the lessons learned from SARS, where there were some quite severe measures introduced. In retrospect, they state, it became clear that some of the strategies were more extensive than necessary to address the public health crisis at hand. The report highlights that, where outcomes are uncertain and potentially catastrophic, liberty-restricting actions may well be justified by values such as solidarity and reciprocity, provided that the restrictions are informed by evidence, proportionate to the threat, carried out humanely and limited to the immediate crisis at hand. At the time of the pandemic, the United Nations (UN) issued a policy brief on the impact of COVID-19 on older people (UN 2020), which stated, "Ensure that visitor policies in residential care facilities, hospitals and hospices balance the protection of others with their need for family and connection." WHO's updated IPC guidance for LTCFs, issued around a year into the pandemic, did seem to use more of the language of compassion. It provided new advice on policies for visitors to and considerations on minimizing the mental and physical health impacts of restrictions and IPC precautions implemented in the context of COVID-19. The guidance acknowledged that lessons learned from implementation and emerging evidence showed that cessation of visiting had a significantly negative impact on the wellbeing of both LTCF residents and their families, along with mental health consequences (WHO 2021). The use of the word visiting here and across other guidance is problematic—a husband entering a care home to spend time with his wife is not a visitor; however, this is not the focus of this chapter.

An important reflection during this period was the "either or" conundrum: IPC or quality of life. One study in the Netherlands stated, "Every day, nursing homes face the dilemma of infection prevention versus allowing personal contact for residents." Perhaps the perceived norm, and as such a prevailing issue, was that IPC is draconian, it is black and white, it is non-negotiable and it ignores the psychosocial. This must be challenged. This is why the statements in the letter were of such importance.

8.6 THE HIERARCHY OF CONTROLS

That the novel coronavirus warranted some "special actions" to stop it spreading from anyone who had it or might have it, to others who were susceptible to getting it, that is, not immune, is not under question. What is under scrutiny is the nature of these "special actions"—also known as IPC. IPC employs an approach based on the five hierarchy of controls framework that includes elimination, substitution, engineering controls, administrative controls and personal protective equipment (PPE) summarised in a training animation launched during the pandemic (NHSE et al. 2021).

REFLECTION EXERCISE

Before reading on, take time to watch the six-minute animation "Every Action Counts—Hierarchy of Controls for Infection Prevention and Control" available on YouTube: www.youtube.com/watch?v=Hj-ZXResT50.

Now you have watched it—think about implementation of each of these controls. Consider the person on the receiving end of each of them—not just a patient or resident of a care or residential home, but the loved ones and the impact these controls might have. How would you communicate with patients and their loved ones to explain the need for each of the controls?

As the video and associated materials explain, the top of the hierarchy is elimination, and examples cited include the use of video or phone consultations rather than in-person, thus eliminating any risk of transmission. COVID-19 testing and symptom screening fall under elimination, the aim being to provide results that can be acted on, for example, a positive test will result in a person isolated from others. Substitution is about replacing the hazard—switching a process or practice so that the hazard is avoided. Cycling to work rather than car sharing is given as an example. Engineering controls are about isolating people from the hazard or containing the hazard. This could mean making changes to the care environment to reduce the spread of COVID-19 such as increasing airflow in places where people with COVID are by opening doors and windows. Another example cited is using barriers or screens to prevent spread from person to person. Administrative control are about changing the way people work. Encouraging people not to have extended periods of close contact, having socially distanced breaks, holding remote meetings. In terms of care delivery, the video acknowledges it's not always possible to keep two metres apart, so administrative and other controls cannot be used for direct care delivery. What is needed for direct care delivery involving close proximity and touch is PPE, described as the last level of control in the hierarchy. The video states that when care involves close contact with a patient with COVID-19, PPE provides an additional barrier—protecting the mucous membranes of the eyes, nose and mouth. For PPE to be effective, it must be worn correctly, with hand hygiene reinforced at the right moments.

8.7 CONSIDERING THE CONSEQUENCES OF ELIMINATION

Turning attention back to care homes (yet equally relevant to hospitals), it appears that for a number of reasons, what happened was a near universal decision to go for the implementation of an extreme form of elimination. People were essentially eliminated from the lives of their loved ones through what became known as "blanket visitor" bans. The focus was on the top of the hierarchy of controls. It is not clear to what extent consideration was given to the psychosocial impact of each of the controls, although the perceived narrative seemed to emerge that the use of video technology limited some of the psychosocial harms associated with elimination. The overt omission of any mention of psychological harms in the hierarchy of controls animation, which is no doubt excellent from a technical perspective, does not come across as person centred.

Back to de-implementation. As each wave of the virus came and went, and "lockdowns" were lifted before being re-imposed, most care homes (and hospitals) continued with elimination. They remained rigidly stuck in the top three of the hierarchy with phrases such as "window visits" becoming normalised and the use of plastic screens and pods and visits encouraged in cars and gardens, even in the freezing cold. Was this a matter of trust? Was it that husbands and wives and daughters and sons and partners and sisters and brothers and friends of 50 years were not trusted with the PPE part of the hierarchy of controls? It certainly seemed that elimination trumped all.

While there are many examples of care homes and hospitals that did everything they possibly could to enable face-to-face interactions and to unite people in a safe way at their most vulnerable moments, there were far too many examples where this was not the case. Dissecting what was behind this is complex. Anecdotal feedback suggests a number of causes at every level of the health system. The guidance does not seem to have overtly addressed the need for discretion and compassionate implementation, or where it did, it was ambiguous and open to misinterpretation. Communication about the guidance from all the different national agencies was often fragmented, leaving those implementing it confused and making decisions that erred on the side of caution. Anecdotal evidence suggests that there was no single voice of leadership nor clear direction from the top. This resulted in an inability to answer questions with clarity and understanding, both from LTCFs and loved ones. Those on the front line were anxious and fearful and required support and permissions that were often missing. Across every level, however, it seemed that for the most part there was a reluctance to ask the questions—how can we solve this problem together so that we can be safe and compassionate? How can we make sure that an 89-year-old lady who may not have many days on this earth left—how can we make sure she can see and hear and feel the presence of her loved ones using these controls to facilitate a safe interaction of what Bialik and Harari (2021) refer to as the non-technological kind? How can we put in place IPC with compassion?

8.8 THE "OH GOD" MOMENT OF THE TWENTY-FIRST CENTURY?

In 1991 Krieger considered the "cruel and crucial lessons" that could and should be learned from the AIDS epidemic and called for vision, resources, and leadership (Krieger 1991). Thirty years later this remains most relevant, but this time in the context of a different infectious disease. Indeed, this chapter started by looking back to a chapter in a previous book and the examples of IPC being used to justify the unjustifiable. In the previous book, we also recalled how some people were treated in the era of HIV and MRSA, citing one colleague who said, "Oh god, what are we doing?" What happened in too many settings across the world during 2020 and 2021 could be the "oh god" moment of the twenty-first century, and in years to come, it will be no surprise if the next generation once again look back in horror at how we treated some of our most vulnerable citizens.

8.9 RECOMMENDATIONS

Informed by these reflections and the lingering aftermath of what happened, there is an opportunity for a new conversation on IPC and compassion, one that ensures measures are always applied in a humane context. The bottom line is that IPC works, and safe IPC practices can be implemented with compassion enabling safe care. As mentioned in a podcast on this subject, a strengthened, compassionate IPC, including how guidance is implemented into practice, could be one of the many positive legacies of COVID-19 (Storr 2021). To fully realise this however will require a number of things to happen, and these are presented here as a series of interrelated recommendations. Actioning these recommendations will ensure that what happened in LTCFs, and other institutions, during the COVID-19 pandemic never happens again.

1. Strengthen IPC leadership and influence in national public health decision-making—it is only by doing this that IPC will influence policymakers, regulators, the media and the public more effectively. When a policymaker stands up on national TV, we want them to speak IPC sense, not IPC nonsense, the same for a scientist, a campaigner, a health leader and a member of the public. This will be a difficult one to crack since it is somewhat outside of the immediate control of IPC, but it can be a goal. The IPC leaders of the future who can nudge this forward may well be reading these words right now.

2. A new movement, compassion-informed IPC, starts today. This includes hardwiring compassion within IPC competencies, which then ripples out into IPC guidance and implementation strategies that communicate the guidance with simple clarity in an easy-to-digest format to those at the "grass roots." The www.enablesafecare.org website, codeveloped by experts, myself included, and a campaign group attempted to do just that. Using the heartbreaking stories from this period to inform future work in this area seems a fitting legacy.

3. Take account of the day-to-day realities of health and social care—learning from some of the pitfalls of previous attempts to hardwire compassion into general nursing care will be key. An evaluation of the national nursing strategy that introduced the 6Cs into the UK revealed "professional anger, distress and resistance to the Compassion in Practice Vision and Strategy" (O'Driscoll et al. 2018). The review highlighted that the programme was viewed as a top-down initiative which did not sufficiently recognise structural constraints on nurses' ability to deliver compassionate care. Collaboration with other professional bodies to ensure compassionate-IPC is not addressed in isolation from the reality of people's work is a must.

4. Frontline practitioners require support in their IPC-related decision-making and communication, particularly around proportionality, discretion, risk communication and application of compassion. Looking back and learning from what happened in the days of AIDS and Ebola will be helpful. It is important not to underestimate the fear that many in health and social care felt in the early days of the COVID-19 pandemic, and IPC practitioners and others can be part of a solution to support a fearful health worker in their role so that a balanced and safe approach ensues. There are excellent examples to be learned from the COVID-19 pandemic, of LTCFs who endeavoured to apply IPC standards with compassion in their efforts to make life bearable for all. IPC practitioners and those interested in the specialty need to be the exemplars, the role models and the champions in this regard.

5. More research on this can be no bad thing. Larson highlighted that each generation looks for their own path, often disregarding the lessons that could be learned from the past (Larson 2022). She cites one example being "the repetition time and again of the same or similar research studies and the publication of articles addressing the same issues that are repeated over and over again across time." Perhaps another positive legacy of the COVID-19 pandemic will be a groundswell of new research on IPC and compassion that can drive a step-change in practice.

Across each of these recommendations is an underlying need to ensure that IPC isn't just about the germ but the person and that IPC advice considers safety and humanity and the sanity of all concerned in equal measure. IPC should not merely be used or misused as an instrument of authority but as a person-centred component of safe and quality health care. A focus on compassion in health care is not new. What seems to be new however is attempting to join the dots between talking about compassion and its relevance to the impact of some IPC practices. IPC guidance doesn't get implemented and interpreted in a microbiology laboratory or a vacuum but in people's real lives and in their real end of lives—it is important to remember this. IPC is a matter of ethics and humanity as well as safety, the ethos of which is to protect people. IPC should never be used as a blunt instrument that in some instances protects people to death.

8.10 REFERENCES

Bialik, M., & Harari, Y. N. (2021, May 27) Mayim Bialik and Yuval Noah Harari in conversation. [video] YouTube www.youtube.com/watch?v=efohpI3sOCI

Cornwell, J. (2014, November 17). Schwartz rounds: Spread 'small acts of kindness' among staff. *Health Service Journal.* www.hsj.co.uk/schwartz-rounds-spread-small-acts-of-kindness-among-staff/5076549.article. Accessed 11 February 2022

Department of Health and NHS Commissioning Board (2012). Compassion in practice. Nursing, midwifery and care staff: Our vision and strategy. www.england.nhs.uk/wp-content/uploads/2012/12/compassion-in-practice.pdf. Accessed 13 February 2022

Francis, R. (2013). *Report of the Mid Staffordshire NHS Foundation Trust Public Inquiry February 2013 Executive Summary. HC 947.* London: The Stationary Office. https://assets.publishing.service.gov.uk/government/uploads/system/uploads/attachment_data/file/279124/0947.pdf

Krieger, N. (1991). Solidarity and AIDS: Introduction. *International Journal of Health Services: Planning, Administration, Evaluation, 21*(3), 505–510. https://doi.org/10.2190/1Q0M-1JJT-3MHU-5CLJ

Larson, E. (2022, February). Looking back to move forward. *American Journal of Infection Control,* 50(2), 123–125. Doi: 10.1016/j.ajic.2021.10.007. PMID: 35101176. www.ajicjournal.org/article/S0196-6553(21)00672-6/fulltext. Accessed 13 February 2022

Martin, G. P., & Dixon-Woods, M. (2014). After mid Staffordshire: From acknowledgement, through learning, to improvement. *BMJ Quality & Safety, 23*(9), 706–708. https://doi.org/10.1136/bmjqs-2014-003359

NHSE, PHE, IPS (2021, March 22). Every action counts—hierarchy of controls for infection prevention and control. YouTube. www.youtube.com/watch?v=Hj-ZXResT50

Norton, W. E., Kennedy, A. E., & Chambers, D. A. (2017). Studying de-implementation in health: An analysis of funded research grants. *Implementation Science, 12*, 144. https://doi.org/10.1186/s13012-017-0655-z.https://implementationscience.biomedcentral.com/articles/10.1186/s13012-017-0655-z#citeas. Accessed 10 February 2022

O'Driscoll, M., Allan, H., Liu, L., Corbett, K., & Serrant, L. (2018). Compassion in practice-Evaluating the awareness, involvement and perceived impact of a national nursing and midwifery strategy amongst healthcare professionals in NHS Trusts in England. *Journal of Clinical Nursing, 27*(5–6), e1097–e1109. https://doi.org/10.1111/jocn.14176

Rubinkam, M. (2021, June 19) 'Protected them to death': Elder-care COVID rules under fire. *The Independent*. www.independent.co.uk/news/protected-them-to-death-eldercare-covid-rules-under-fire-new-york-pennsylvania-rochester-america-cincinnati-b1869032.html

Storr, J. (2016). Just infection prevention and control. In P. Elliott, J. Storr, & A. Jeanes (Eds.), *Infection Prevention and Control: Perceptions and Perspectives*. Boca Raton: Taylor and Francis.

Storr, J. (2021). Compassion and infection prevention—not mutually exclusive. Infection control matters: Discussions on infection prevention. *Podcast*. Wednesday August 18, 2021. https://infectioncontrolmatters.podbean.com/e/compassion-and-infection-prevention-not-mutually-exclusive/

Storr, J. et al. (2020, October 16). Open letter: Infection prevention and control should never be at the expense of compassionate care. *Nursing Times*. www.nursingtimes.net/opinion/open-letter-infection-prevention-and-control-should-never-be-at-the-expense-of-compassionate-care-16–10–2020/. Accessed 13 February 2022

Storr, J., Kilpatrick, C., & Vassallo, A. (2021). Safe infection prevention and control practices with compassion—A positive legacy of COVID-19. *American Journal of Infection Control, 49*(3), 407–408. https://doi.org/10.1016/j.ajic.2020.12.016

Suárez-González, A., & Storr, J. (2021, July 15). Enforced restrictions to care home access—unfair, unnecessary, and harmful. *The BMJ Opinion*. https://blogs.bmj.com/bmj/2021/07/15/enforced-restrictions-to-care-home-access-unfair-unnecessary-and-harmful/. Accessed 13 February 2022

Treciak, S., & Mazarelli, A. (2019). *Compassionomics: The Revolutionary Scientific Evidence That Caring Makes a Difference*. Florida, US: Studer Group.

United Nations Policy Brief: The Impact of COVID-19 on older persons May 2020 www.un.org/development/desa/ageing/wp-content/uploads/sites/24/2020/05/COVID-Older-persons.pdf. Accessed 13 February 2022

WHO (2015). *Global Health Ethics*. Key Issues. https://apps.who.int/iris/bitstream/handle/10665/164576/9789240694033_eng.pdf?sequence=1&isAllowed=y. Accessed 13 February 2022

World Health Organization. (2021, January 8). *Infection Prevention and Control Guidance for Long-Term Care Facilities in the Context of COVID-19: Interim Guidance*. World Health Organization. https://apps.who.int/iris/handle/10665/338481. Accessed 13 February 2022

Why Do We Choose to Work in Infection Prevention and Control?

9

Annette Jeanes

Contents

> There is nothing more difficult to take in hand, more perilous to conduct, or more uncertain in its success, than to take the lead in the introduction of a new order of things.
>
> Niccolo Machiavelli

9.1 INTRODUCTION

The delivery of an optimal and effective infection prevention and control (IPC) service is contingent on several factors, including the support and contribution of society and healthcare organisations (Brannigan et al. 2009). Some individuals choose to take on roles

DOI: 10.1201/9781003379393-11

which lead and deliver this speciality, whilst others are content to act as champions and role models. This chapter examines some of the reasons why they make this choice, some of the challenges they face and why they continue to work in this area. The examples used are from the author's experiences of working as an IPC specialist.

9.2 ROLE VALUE

Undertaking roles which aim to prevent harm can be challenging (Thacker & MacKenzie 2003). Those making the efforts to reduce danger and prevent harm are often distanced in time and location from those benefiting from the planning, education, investment, and actions previously taken. Consequently, the value and contribution of these roles may not be fully recognised, particularly if no harm occurs. In roles such as fire prevention and road safety, it could be argued that the dangers and the potential for harm is relatively easy to explain as examples are regularly in the media and the importance of such prevention is widely recognised. In contrast, the prevention of infection often involves dealing with an invisible danger which may take time to develop or emerge as a problem and requires actions and behaviours which may be perceived as impeding efforts to deliver care. It may be particularly difficult to justify this service or advice if there is a lack of awareness of infections or their impact. The work of Ignaz Semmelweis exemplifies this challenge.

Ironically, the success of preventing and controlling infection and the absence or reduction of outbreaks or infections may also undermine the perceived need for infection prevention and control expertise and specialist roles. Though, the regular emergence of novel organisms, significant variants, treatment resistant microorganism and circumstances which enable the development and transmission of organisms, for example, disasters, poor hygiene, antibiotic overuse, have ensured that infection prevention and control expertise and advice is constantly in demand (McCloskey et al. 2014).

The perceived value of the IPC role may fluctuate, and in times of crisis such as outbreaks or pandemics, the role is seen as crucial, whilst during less difficult times, justification may be required for the continuance of posts or funding. This may be particularly problematic following on from a period such as a pandemic or outbreak, when the basics of infection controls are widely recognised and just about everyone becomes an infection expert!

There is evidence that compliant ICP behaviour and attitudes wane over time and revert to the baseline level in most instances (Kirkland & Craig 2011). This is despite the intermittent panics when an infectious disease or infection is perceived to be a problem but is not a threat (Pappas et al. 2009). Consequently, the sustained input of ICP education and advice is essential to allay fears and sustain compliance with required controls.

9.3 MOTIVATION

The need to keep reminding a potentially disinterested audience "not to forget the basics" can be frustrating when the dangers appear to have passed, and some may question why anyone does the job. The reason people undertake an IPC role varies, and it should be acknowledged that not everyone actively chooses this role or responsibility as some do it as part of another job or because of necessity.

The motivation to undertake this role may be understood in terms of the human needs described by Maslow (1943, 1954) and range from the need for a job to provide food and shelter and the psychological and self-fulfilment needs of belongingness, relationships, esteem, respect, and prestige. Maslow's theory was criticised and revised in his lifetime (Kachalla 2014) as it was based on a limited sample and did not reflect some of the complexities of motivation such as external, internal, material and nonmaterial factors. It is now recognised that understanding motivation is complex and many theories exist.

Underlying motivation may also be explained in terms of self-determination theory (Deci & Ryan 2008) within the constructs of autonomous and controlled motivation (Tam et al. 2019). Autonomous motivation reflects the values, experiences, interests and goals of individuals (Koestner et al. 2008). This form of motivation is related to life experience, education, beliefs and may be evident, for example, in qualities such as honesty, resilience and commitment, influences, preferences, trust and risk-taking. This may include taking on challenges such as preventing harm, keeping people safe and the potential to lead and make changes.

Controlled motivation relates to the external and internal pressures and rewards experienced by the person whilst in the role and organisation. External pressures include a pay, career progression and status, whilst internal rewards include job satisfaction, the respect of others and avoiding the consequence of failure. It may be difficult to unpick the type of motivation responsible for choices, but autonomous motivation is more likely to persist whilst controlled motivation may wane once the external and internal pressures cease (Grant 2008).

The motivation to do the role is also influenced by the individual's understanding of what the role involves and how this fits their needs. Some may interpret the role as one which primarily focuses on the speciality of infection prevention and control and are attracted to less responsibility for the routine hands-on care of patients and more opportunities for flexible working. Others may enjoy the autonomy or the opportunity to do a job which is unpredictable and continuously evolving and presenting new challenges (Chung-Yan 2010; Conway et al. 2013). Equally some may be attracted to the structure and continuity of auditing, collecting data, undertaking research, writing reports, teaching and enabling others to optimise practice, which is often part of the role.

9.4 ORGANISATION

Whilst the motivation and intentions of practitioners may vary, the expectations and responsibilities of the role also differs in organisations and cultures and continues to evolve (Conway et al. 2013). These differences may be affected by organisational strategy, vision, memory, workload, funding, environment and conditions. Consequently, the underlying motivation and intention of IPC practitioners may not at times align with the expectations and objectives of the organisation (Kyratsis et al. 2019), which may significantly affect job satisfaction.

This is particularly problematic when the organisational culture or strategic vision does not prioritise patient safety values, does not perceive infection control as a safety issue or does not recognise the value of infection prevention and control input at strategic and operational levels. This may undermine the motives of IPC professionals, and the barriers encountered may lead to dissatisfaction and despondency. This may be may evident in situations such as when there is a need to close a service because of an outbreak, as priorities such as maintaining a vital service, generating income and minimising reputational damage may come into conflict with the infection control advice and requirements. Other examples include how the organisation responds to noncompliance with infection control policies of senior staff and reporting an error or performance data, which highlights failure.

The organisation or managers may also not recognise the effort and value of the ICP practitioner and/or team when they are efficient and effective. Examples include the development of a policy, plan or information prior to the emergence of the problem, provision of education and training to ensure staff are prepared and know what to do or the additional unpaid working hours. It is not uncommon for IPC to feel disgruntled that their work is often invisible to the organisation and that their efforts are not recognised.

9.5 ROLE CONFLICT

There may be role conflict (Schuler & Aldag 1977) as the IPC practitioner may be required to undertake several roles, such as subject matter expert, researcher, manager, director, budget holder and work across departments or organisations. This can be difficult to achieve and may contribute to confusion and ambiguity about the role both for the individual and others within the workplace. There may be a balancing act, for example, between meeting organisational expectations and priorities, responding to queries, leading a team, promoting safety, utilizing evidence-based practice, expediency, maintaining good working relationships and having a life outside work.

The specialist knowledge, skills and experience which is required to work as an IPC practitioner may at times be insufficient to operate effectively within a complex organisation or unfamiliar situation. The trust, confidence and support of colleagues and of key decision-makers is essential to undertake the role successfully, and being clear about what is required to do the job well will hopefully be welcomed. Expectations of "hitting the ground running" or having an immediate and definitive answer in every situation that presents is unrealistic as sometimes a period of reflection, review of the evidence and discussion are needed before decisions are made or advice is given. Explaining that answers are not straightforward may cause disappointment and stress to both parties.

9.6 DON'T SHOOT THE MESSENGER

The IPC role may often involve giving messages or feedback which people may not like or want and may cause tension or conflict (Baron 1988). Whilst it is preferable to tread carefully and work with people to improve performance and quality, sometimes it is necessary to intervene to prevent harm. Examples range from reminding someone to clean their hands between a dirty and aseptic task, insisting that a patient is isolated to prevent transmission, asking a manager to send home a healthcare worker with diarrhoea and vomiting when the department is short-staffed and busy. In such instances the presence of clear policies and guidance with managerial support is essential.

Sometimes there may be an expectation of "turning a blind eye" or making exceptions, which can be problematic, for example, "The wards are full, can we temporarily double up in patient bed spaces?" "Do we really need to reprocess rather than just wipe this endoscope after it fell on the floor as it's a long list and will cause delays or cancellations?" "Can't we stop the screening as there are no isolation facilities left?" The recipient's response to an undesired answer may be to ask someone else until the preferred response is achieved, alternately "pressure" may be applied to achieve the favoured answer. This can undermine the confidence of the IPC practitioner, who may find themselves seeking allies to back up their response, lowering their standards or using tactics to avoid answering questions which are problematic.

9.7 BULLYING AND INTIMIDATION

Those ICPs who are motivated by career progression beyond infection prevention and control may favour appeasement rather than standing their ground, and sometimes a negotiated compromise is a rational response to a difficult situation. An alternative is to persist in responding truthfully, but this has consequences as this may lead to the development of a negative perception of the person and/or role within the organisation. This can lead to bullying of the IPC practitioner by undermining opinion, exclusion from information, lack of recognition of effort, pressure to achieve unachievable deadlines and exclusion from opportunities (Rayner & Hoel 1997).

Bullying is common in health care (Carter et al. 2013), and in many professions and organisations, the expectation is to "suck it up" and not complain (Quine 1999). The lack of support of organisations in such situations has been termed "organisational betrayal" (Khrais 2018), which increases stress and decreases job satisfaction (Brewer et al. 2020). The organisation may be blind to the effects on individuals as it is an established part of the culture, but it will impact on performance and retention (Pope & Burnes 2013).

IPC are particularly vulnerable to a lack of recognition that bullying is occurring as they may operate across and outside the established organisational structures and behaviours, and responses may not be noticed. In addition, they are dependent on others to accept choices and practices which may be unpopular, and therefore the ICP may be reluctant to alienate colleagues who respond negatively. It is recognised that identifying and reporting a significant problem can lead to victimisation of the "whistle-blower" and the practice of "gaslighting" where self-doubt is induced when the response of those in power is to deny there is a problem (Ahern 2018). In some organisations bad practice becomes the norm, and this "cultural entrapment" (Weick & Sutcliffe 2003) rationalises and justifies this behaviour, which makes challenging and changing practice difficult. Indeed, the IPC practitioner may be identified as deviant or bullying if they persist in challenging the organisation.

9.8 JOB SATISFACTION

The issues outlined previously are not unique to IPC roles, but despite such impediments, many find the IPC role satisfying and fulfilling, particularly as the desire to prevent harm is a powerful motivator (Grant & Hofmann 2011). The benefit for others is evident when there is a positive and open response to preventable tragedies and mistakes, which drive improvements and initiatives (Tanne 2006).

It is particularly satisfying to undertake a preventative role whilst working in an organisation which has a culture of safety and learning (Egan et al. 2004) and with the support of leaders (Larson et al. 2007). Other factors which can increase satisfaction, support motivation and make the job easier are sufficient resources, collaborative working, teamwork (Rafferty et al. 2001), good communication, empowerment, engagement, working for a common goal (Bion et al. 2013) and recognition of efforts (Danish & Usman 2010). The lack of these factors may decrease job satisfaction and consequently motivation (Kian et al. 2014) in even the most enthusiastic, optimistic and altruistic.

In the experience of the author, some individuals are unable to sustain the motivation and passion to do the job effectively, whilst others become obsessed with aspects of the work such as writing policies, auditing, going to meetings, ventilation monitoring or cleaning. This can affect the workload and experience of others in the team and has implications for how the IPC service functions and is perceived. Whilst flexibility and resilience are essential qualities of IPCs, carrying the workload and responsibilities of burnt-out or dysfunctional members of the team affects job satisfaction. An honest conversation with the individual may be difficult but is preferable to immediately escalating concerns to managers.

9.9 SPECIALISM

An aspect of this and similar specialist roles relates to being a specialist, knowing more than nonspecialists about the subject and being one of a group of specialists. The evolving nature of the speciality, challenges and rarity of specialist knowledge and experience have led to the development of societies and groups of specialists, to support and share knowledge and experience.

Many specialities develop their own terminology and subcultures which are exclusive to members or others with similar interests, which is beneficial as it increases the dissemination of knowledge within the group and support to people who may work in isolation. Within such groups, an elite emerge over time (Cheng et al. 2013; Henrich & Gil-White 2001) who are valued for their specialist knowledge and experience and act as role models. Motivation to undertake the IPC role may be influenced by the rewards of membership and status and influence from such a group. It is also possible that a member may be ascribed power and influence within such a group, which is not available in their own role or organisation. This has been described previously in, for example, trade union steward roles, where people gain prestige, power, recognition and deference externally rather than in their day job (Drucker 2017).

9.10 CONCLUSION

Undertaking an infection prevention and control role is challenging. The ICP may be in the spotlight during outbreaks or infection-related incidents, but much of the day-to-day prevention-based work may not be noticed if it is effective. The constant changes in expectations, evidence and practice can require considerable input behind the scenes to remain competent and credible. The delivery of unpopular messages and the consequences of persisting to prioritise infection prevention and patent safety can be difficult.

Despite all the potentially negative aspects of the role, participating in the delivery of infection prevention and control can be interesting, fulfilling and stimulating, delivering considerable benefits. Organisational leadership, team support, specialist groupings or societies and the help of colleagues all contribute to job satisfaction. Whilst the enthusiasm to continue to prompt people to clean their hands or not to wear disposable gloves for every task may sometimes wane, it can be inspiring and at times humbling to see the outcomes of efforts to prevent avoidable harm and keep people safe.

9.11 REFLECTIVE EXERCISE

1. What motivates you to work in this speciality?
2. What would improve your job satisfaction?
3. List three healthcare practitioners who have improved their infection control practice because of your influence or input
4. What are your personal goals in undertaking your infection control role?

9.12 REFERENCES

Ahern K. Institutional betrayal and gaslighting. *The Journal of Perinatal & Neonatal Nursing.* 2018;32:59–65.

Baron RA. Negative effects of destructive criticism: Impact on conflict, self-efficacy, and task performance. *Journal of Applied Psychology.* 1988;73:199–207.

Bion J, Richardson A, Hibbert P, The Matching Michigan Collaboration & Writing Committee, et al 'Matching Michigan': A 2-year stepped interventional programme to minimise central venous catheter-blood stream infections in intensive care units in England. *BMJ Quality & Safety.* 2013;22:110–23.

Brannigan ET, Murray E, Holmes A. Where does infection control fit into a hospital management structure? *Journal of Hospital Infection.* 2009;73:392–6.

Brewer KC, Oh KM, Kitsantas P, Zhao X. Workplace bullying among nurses and organizational response: An online cross-sectional study. *Journal of Nursing Management.* 2020;28:148–56.

Carter M, Thompson N, Crampton P, Morrow G, Burford B, Gray C, Illing J. Workplace bullying in the UK NHS: A questionnaire and interview study on prevalence, impact and barriers to reporting. *BMJ Open.* 2013;3(6):e002628.

Cheng JT, Tracy JL, Foulsham T, Kingstone A, Henrich J. Two ways to the top: Evidence that dominance and prestige are distinct yet viable avenues to social rank and influence. *Journal of Personality and Social Psychology.* 2013;104:103.

Chung-Yan GA. The nonlinear effects of job complexity and autonomy on job satisfaction, turnover, and psychological well-being. *Journal of Occupational Health Psychology.* 2010;15:237.

Conway LJ, Raveis VH, Pogorzelska-Maziarz M, Uchida M, Stone PW, Larson EL. Tensions inherent in the evolving role of the infection preventionist. *American Journal of Infection Control.* 2013;41:959–64.

Danish RQ, Usman A. Impact of reward and recognition on job satisfaction and motivation: An empirical study from Pakistan. *International Journal of Business and Management.* 2010;5:159.

Deci EL, Ryan RM. Self-determination theory: A macrotheory of human motivation, development, and health. *Canadian Psychology/Psychologie Canadienne.* 2008;49:182–5.

Drucker PF. *The New Society: The Anatomy of Industrial Order.* Oxford: Routledge; 2017.

Egan TM, Yang B, Bartlett KR. The effects of organizational learning culture and job satisfaction on motivation to transfer learning and turnover intention. *Human Resource Development Quarterly.* 2004;15:279–301.

Grant AM. Does intrinsic motivation fuel the prosocial fire? Motivational synergy in predicting persistence, performance, and productivity. *Journal of Applied Psychology.* 2008;93:48.

Grant AM, Hofmann DA. It's not all about me: Motivating hand hygiene among health care professionals by focusing on patients. *Psychological Science.* 2011;22:1494–9.

Henrich J, Gil-White FJ. The evolution of prestige: Freely conferred deference as a mechanism for enhancing the benefits of cultural transmission. *Evolution and Human Behavior.* 2001;22:165–96.

Kachalla B. Review of the role of motivation on employee performance. *Mediterranean Journal of Social Sciences.* 2014;5:39.

Khrais H, Higazee MZ, Khalil M, Wahab SD. Impact of organizational support on nursing job stressors: A comparative study. *Health Science Journal.* 2018;12:1–6.

Kian TS, Yusoff WF, Rajah S. Job satisfaction and motivation: What are the difference among these two. *European Journal of Business and Social Sciences.* 2014;3:94–102.

Kirkland K, Craig SR. *A Qualitative Analysis of Facilitators and Barriers to Hand Hygiene Improvement at New Hampshire Hospitals during a Statewide Hand Hygiene Campaign. Foundation for Healthy Communities.* Concord, NH: Foundation for Healthy Communities; 2011 Nov.

Koestner R, Otis N, Powers TA, Pelletier L, Gagnon H. Autonomous motivation, controlled motivation, and goal progress. *Journal of Personality*. 2008;76:1201–30.

Kyratsis Y, Ahmad R, Iwami M, Castro-Sánchez E, Atun R, Holmes AH. A multilevel neo-institutional analysis of infection prevention and control in English hospitals: Coerced safety culture change? *Sociology of Health & Illness*. 2019;41:1138–58.

Larson EL, Quiros D, Lin SX. Dissemination of the CDC's hand hygiene guideline and impact on infection rates. *American Journal of Infection Control*. 2007;35:666–75.

Maslow AH. A theory of human motivation. *Psychological Review*. 1943;50:370–96.

Maslow AH. *Motivation and Personality*. New York: Harper and Row; 1954.

McCloskey B, Dar O, Zumla A, Heymann DL. Emerging infectious diseases and pandemic potential: Status quo and reducing risk of global spread. *The Lancet Infectious Diseases*. 2014;14:1001–10.

Pappas G, Kiriaze IJ, Giannakis P, Falagas ME. Psychosocial consequences of infectious diseases. *Clinical Microbiology and Infection*. 2009;15:743–7.

Pope R, Burnes B. A model of organisational dysfunction in the NHS. *Journal of Health Organization and Management*. 2013 Oct 28;27:676–97.

Quine L. Workplace bullying in NHS community trust: Staff questionnaire survey. *BMJ*. 1999;318:228–32.

Rafferty AM, Ball J, Aiken LH. Are teamwork and professional autonomy compatible, and do they result in improved hospital care? *BMJ Quality & Safety*. 2001;10(Suppl 2):ii32–7.

Rayner C, Hoel H. A summary review of literature relating to workplace bullying. *Journal of Community & Applied Social Psychology*. 1997;7:181–91.

Schuler RS, Aldag RJ, Brief AP. Role conflict and ambiguity: A scale analysis. *Organizational Behavior and Human Performance*. 1977;20:111–28.

Tam AY, Baharun R, Sulaiman Z. Motivation in health behaviour: Role of autonomous and controlled motivation. *Indian Journal of Public Health*. 2019;10:909.

Tanne JH. Can stories of personal tragedy spark a healthcare revolution? *BMJ*. 2006;333:924.

Thacker SB, MacKenzie EJ. Preface: The role of the epidemiologist in injury prevention and control—an unmet challenge. *Epidemiologic Reviews*. 2003;25:1–2.

Weick KE, Sutcliffe KM. Hospitals as cultures of entrapment: A re-analysis of the Bristol royal infirmary. *California Management Review*. 2003;45:73–84.

PART 3

Real World Perspectives

Human Factors Engineering in Infection Prevention and Control

10

Hugo Sax

Contents

10.1 WHY HUMAN FACTORS ENGINEERING COULD BRIDGE THE INFECTION PREVENTION AND CONTROL GAP BETWEEN SCIENCE AND BEHAVIOUR

Overall, 30 to 70% of today's healthcare-associated infections are still preventable due to difficulties to consistently apply evidence-based infection prevention measures—despite

DOI: 10.1201/9781003379393-13

decades of efforts (Schreiber et al. 2018). There is an obvious reason why this is such a "hard problem." Microorganisms are invisible, and infections manifest themselves with latency, depriving healthcare providers (HCP) of the behaviour-motivating experiential feedback. Moreover, most preventative actions carry a very small infectious risk when skipped by individuals. The risk becomes only relevant on a statistical level. Yet humans are captivated by current emotional events and the next task at hand, a trait resulting from 200,000 years of evolution in an environment beyond their control. In the last centuries, however, we increasingly live in human-made environments. This provides us with both the opportunity and the accountability for an informed and deliberate design. This is what human factors and ergonomics (HF/E) is about, and its potential to add value to IPC is ripe for exploitation.

10.2 HUMAN FACTORS AS A KNOWLEDGEBASE AND A DISCIPLINE—A LITTLE BIT OF HISTORY

The first mention of ergonomics, a term synonymous with HF/E, in 1857 is credited to Wojciech Jastrzebowski, a Polish scientist and inventor (Jastrzebowski 2000). Yet it was not until the 1940s when many pilots died due to latent errors in aircraft design that HF/E saw increasing application. The discipline was further consolidated in the 1950s and 1960s (Meister 2018) with the foundation of the Ergonomics Research Society in 1949 in the UK (Browne et al. 1950) that evolved into the Chartered Institute of Ergonomics and Human Factors (www.ergonomics.org.uk), the International Ergonomics Association in England in 1959 (Karwowski 2021, https://iea.cc) and the Human Factors and Ergonomics Society in 1957 in the USA (www.hfes.org). HF/E grew from a platform of interdisciplinary exchange between psychologists and engineers into a science, practice and profession, integrating a growing number of knowledge fields (Meister 2018).

The term HF/E is double-edged. It is often misread as to focus on correcting people's proneness to error. "Sociotechnical Systems Engineering for Humans" might be a more accurate term but somewhat unwieldly. The International Ergonomics Association reflects this broader system's view in their HF/E definition:

> Ergonomics (or Human Factors) is the scientific discipline concerned with the understanding of interactions among humans and other elements of a system, and the profession that applies theory, principles, data and methods to design in order to optimize human well-being and overall system performance.
>
> (Human Factors and Ergonomics Society 2021)

In his wide-read book *The Human Factor* Vicente delivers a simple visualisation of HF/E potential for a broad application as a "Human-Tech Ladder" (Vicente 2004). The two side rails represent the human and the tech components of sociotechnical systems.

The steps symbolise the physical, psychological, team, organisational and political level of HF/E application. The application of HF/E to the organisational level is also called macroergonomics (Carayon et al. 2013). However, it is this wide scope and intrinsic inter-disciplinarity that also continues to challenge its identity as a science and a profession (Meister 2018).

Sociotechnical systems are inherently complex. They display specific features such as non-linearity, emergence, spontaneous order, adaptation and feedback loops (Staiger 2016). They are composed of subsystems that react to context according to inner rules and change the context for other subsystems (Plsek & Greenhalgh 2001). These characteristics challenge traditional engineering approaches that build only on central control and standardization and entirely overlook the potential of human adaptivity and creativity.

10.3 MENTAL MODELS AND OTHER COGNITIVE RESOURCES

Among the many human features to be considered by HF/E, the concept of mental models is especially useful. According to this model of human cognition, we have a "small-scale model" of the external reality in our mind (Johnson-Laird 1983, 2006; Mental Models Global Laboratory 2021). These models deliver an actionable understanding of the reality around us based on cues in the incoming stream of sensory information. How mental models work can be taken from Figure 10.1. Mental models do not necessarily have to be entirely correct to be useful. As an example, the throttle of modern motorbikes controls the engine regime electronically and not by a physical wire anymore. A rider can ride her bike perfectly well while still mistakenly imagining the traditional steel wire moving a valve on the carburettor. In other situations, however, inadequate mental models can trigger misunderstandings in communication and erroneous actions. The firm belief of the captain of KLM flight 4805 that he was cleared for takeoff made him ignore the warnings by his copilots and led to the collision with another airplane on Tenerife Airport that killed 583 people (KLM-PAA. Joint Report 1978) [16]. Recent neuroscience research confirms the idea of a top-down construction of human reality in a radical way as "controlled hallucination" (Anil 2020). These human factors are considered by asking: "What are the mental models of the concerned (various) humans who will be active in the future sociotechnical system?"

Two other relevant cognitive human traits concern attention and recall (Branaghan et al. 2021). Humans can only focus on one thing at a time. This is gloriously demonstrated by the famous "The invisible gorilla" experiment (www.youtube.com/watch?v=IGQmdoK_ZfY) (Chabris & Simons 2010). The same can be tested in Figure 10.1. The limited reliability of human memory has led to the idea of "knowledge in the world," for example, in the form of checklists.

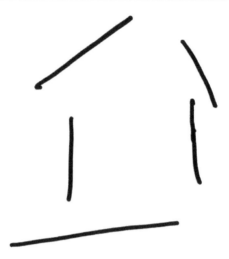

FIGURE 10.1   Mental model self-experiment

Legend for Figure 10.1. Experiment: Look at this figure and say what you see. This experiment provides an experience of our conceptual thinking and projecting of concepts or mental models onto (in this case, visual) sensory input. Try to switch back and forth between seeing a house versus seeing five independent lines (if you manage at all). You will notice that it is impossible to focus your attention on both at the same time.

10.4 HUMAN FACTORS ENGINEERING METHODS

Imagine you want to use an elevator. You would obviously like to intuitively press the right button and be reassured that the elevator is on its way. A systems view of this situation would picture the subsystem "human" and the subsystem "elevator" exchanging information through the interface "elevator control panel" to execute the transport task. The control panel tells you where to press. By pressing, you tell the elevator system to send an elevator. The elevator confirms and ideally updates you how long you must still wait. However, as we have all experienced, these panels are often poorly designed and, let's say, fail to consider the intuitive human assumption that "What belongs together, goes (spatially) together," as illustrated in Figure 10.2. This example of a human-technology interface shall serve as an illustration for the following discussion of HF/E methods.

HF/E offers a wide array of dedicated tools for systems analysis and design (Stanton 2022). They include methods for data collection, physical and cognitive task analysis, process charting, human error identification and accident analysis, situation awareness assessment, mental workload assessment, team assessment, interface analysis, design, performance time prediction and their integration (Stanton et al. 2013). These tools typically use quantitative and qualitative methods and cover physiologic, cognitive and organisational aspects (Karwowski 2021). Cognitive work analysis (CWA), a demanding but flexible method to assess and describe sociotechnical systems, may serve as one commonly used example (Vicente 1999). These toolsets are part of the HF/E curricula at bachelor, master and PhD level and represent the professional asset of well-trained HF/E professionals.

Hollnagel (2017), however, warns against an overly theoretical approach and suggests a minimal set of principles that are crucial for practical purposes. Here are some of my fundamentals. Everyone involved in the design process has to understand the messy

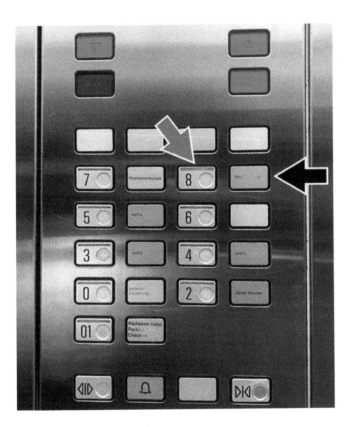

FIGURE 10.2   Elevator interface with a latent error

Legend for Figure 10.2. This is an elevator control panel at the Airport Zurich-Kloten, Switzerland. The building harbours the Airport Medical Centre (AMC) on the eighth floor. The writing on the indication tag (back arrow) is almost gone, showing how many people wrongly pressed on the tag instead of on the control button marked by the floor number 8 (pink arrow). This is a typical "latent error" in the design of the control panel going against the human assumption that "what belongs together goes together." Someone must have realised this design flaw and tried to fix it by guiding the users by marking the true control button with pink colour (pink arrow). Such "patches" are frequent and can point to an underlying design problem.

"work-as-done" at the sharp end instead of "work-as-imagined." To this end, both questioning and observations of those doing the work are necessary since they usually don't consciously monitor their own behaviour. We found video-reflexive ethnography a very useful method in an IPC context, where the two aspects are combined (Iedema et al. 2015). People are video-taped during a certain activity and then asked to comment on their cognitive and emotional process while watching the video-feed. Design-thinking, now often used in industry, offers methods to improve the usability of products (Altman et al. 2018). This iterative method starts with as many uncensored ideas as possible and then how to select the best one(s) via co-creation, making errors early, prototyping, bias towards action and involving future users effectively. Furthermore, there is value in enlarging and tightening the boundaries around the problem at the outset of a design task to determine the right fit. Exemplarily, in the elevator case in the previous section, it would not be the same thing to ask "How do I create the best possible interface between users and an elevator?" versus "How do people get from one level to a desired other level in the building?" or as opposed to "What would a building look like to make navigation most easy?" In addition, I find the system analogy of a riverbed in which water flows downwards simple but powerful. This analogy transports two major ideas. First, the system structure determines its behaviour. This is reflected in the hierarchy of intervention effectiveness by the Institute for Safe Medication Practices spanning from training via checklists to forcing functions from least to most effective (Cafazzo & St-Cyr 2012). While clinicians usually believe in readily changing the behaviour of HCPs through training to improve quality and safety, changes to deeper structures are usually more successful and sustainable. Second, complex systems tend to operate at minimum required energy. Humans always find workarounds that facilitate their tasks. Such workarounds are often necessary to get the work done but can also jeopardise safety. In any case, any design should anticipate this and already minimise necessary efforts to get the job done from the start. And finally, as the elevator control panel shows, interfaces should match the users' mental models and show what is expected and what is going on.

10.5 HUMAN FACTORS IN HEALTH CARE

In 1930 Frank and Lilian Gilbreth, an American research couple at the origin of the "scientific management" movement, studied surgical teams using film and aimed at improving patient safety through standardisation (Baumgart et al. 2009). They introduced the technique of "read backs" during surgical interventions. When the surgeon asks for a "scalpel" the "scrub nurse" would hand it over, equally voicing "scalpel." In a similar vein, standardised checklists have since become standard in surgery albeit over 70 years later! They are, however, only useful if adapted to their context of use (Schmutz et al. 2014; Chaparro et al. 2019). This underlines the evolution from standardization to a complex systems approach.

The idea of HF/E has found a foothold in health care since the late 1990s. The seminal report by the Institute of Medicine on error and error prevention in medicine "To err is human" in 2000 supported the very powerful HF/E idea of "latent errors" that can be hidden in all layers of healthcare systems from physical object to communication and institutional organisation (Kohn et al. 2000). The report suggested to "respect human limits in the design process" by "designing jobs for safety, avoiding reliance on memory, and simplifying and standardizing work processes" (Kohn 2000). More recently, the World Health Organization (WHO) promotes HF/E as a part of their patient safety curriculum (Walton et al. 2010). In parallel, the HF/E community has discovered health care as a target industry. For example, the US Human Factors and Ergonomics Society now organises an annual conference on HF/E in health care with five tracks, "Digital health," "Education and simulation," "Hospital environment," "Medical and drug delivery devices" and "Patient safety research and initiatives" and made many other contributions to health care (Mouloua et al. 2021). A textbook edited by Pascale Carayon provides a large overview of HF/E benefits and applications in health care and patient safety (Carayon 2011), covering macroergonomics, organisational design, information technology and interfaces, telemedicine, human error, and interventions. A widely applied HF/E-inspired model of health care is the Systems Engineering Initiative for Patient Safety (SEIPS) (Xie & Carayon 2015). Following Donabedian's structure-process-outcome logic (Donabedian 1978), the model proposed a component "work system" made of people, environment and tools, a component "processes" and a component "outcomes" (Carayon et al. 2006, 2020; Holden et al. 2013). On the regulatory side, the International Organisation for Standardization (ISO) issued the ISO 26800 norm that describe the general approach, principles and concepts to ergonomic design covering dimensions such as "an ergonomics approach to design shall be human-centred" or "the target population shall be identified and described" (www.sciencedirect.com/book/9780128024218/designing-for-human-reliability). The FDA issued guidance for the healthcare industry to support manufacturers in improving the design of devices to minimise potential use errors and resulting harm (U.S. Department of Health and Human Services, Food and Drug Administration 2016).

10.6 HUMAN FACTORS IN INFECTION PREVENTION AND CONTROL

The uptake of HF/E by IPC has been more hesitant despite over ten years of advocacy. In their excellent 2010 overview paper, Anderson et al. argue that HF/E would be of special benefit to IPC because of the specific challenges of the invisible infectious agents (Anderson et al. 2010). They promote means to make the invisible immediately tangible by fluorescence dye to mimic microorganisms, simulators to train aseptic handling, real-time reporting of cases of healthcare-acquired infections to overcome latency. They also address the benefits of smart products, patient room design and immersive evaluation of the work environment. Other review and advocacy papers have followed (Storr et al. 2013; Pennathur & Herwaldt 2017; Clack & Sax 2017; Jacob et al. 2018; Patel & Kallen 2018; Drews et al. 2019). In 2013, Storr et al. called for an increased capacity and capability of HF/E in IPC and suggest a root and branch review of IPC measures through an

HF/E lens. Pennathur and Herwaldt (2017) literature review of explicit applications of HF/E to IPC have found that "the most significant gap pertains to the limited use and application of formal HF/E tools and methods" and ask for a more holistic approach to the system and system component interaction. Jacob et al. (2018) address hand hygiene, environmental cleaning, personal protective equipment, emergency preparedness, devices and isolation precautions. They propose a larger systems approach and refer to the SEIPS model as a valuable tool for this. They also suggest simplifying care work-flows to better understand why processes fail, how errors can be reduced and efficiency increased. In the most recent review, Drews et al. (2019) describe HF/E solutions and opportunities for IPC challenges such hand hygiene, PPE use and central line associated bloodstream infections. They identify the following areas of beneficial contribution of HF/E to IPC:

(1) development/application of conceptual frameworks of human performance, (2) improved understanding of HCP cognitive processes (e.g., individual and shared mental models), (3) simplification or redesign of workflows, (4) improvement of equipment design, (5) development/optimization of standardized training programs and requirements, (6) elimination of communication/guidelines ambiguity, (7) task-based improvements of the built environment and standardization of equipment placement within and across facilities, and (8) improvements of organizational safety climate.

A quasi-systematic literature search for the purpose of this chapter yielded 85 publications with a marked increase in numbers since 2020, mostly due to the SARS-CoV-2 pandemic (Figure 10.3). Some authors are noticeable for their scientific output. Original investigations reported evaluations in 35 cases, interventions in 14 cases, and both in 4 cases. Thirty-two were reviews, thought papers, or editorials. There is no comparative study to test the value of an HF/E approach against any other initiative. It must be kept in mind, however, that practical engineering projects are not necessarily published in the scientific literature, potentially leading to publication bias. Many publications had to be excluded because they used the term "human factors" solely to address human behaviour.

An example of a holistic systems engineering approach was the Designing Out Medical Error (DOME) project (Norris et al. 2013). In a multidisciplinary collaboration, clinicians, psychologists, economists, and designers set priorities based on a failure mode and effects analysis (FMEA) and produced optimised layouts and tools through observations, codesign techniques, simulations, prototyping and testing. An example of tool engineering and evaluation is the work of Drews et al. (2017). Iterative analysis and design led to a maintenance kit for central lines that integrates a checklist with a "support" that holds all necessary items in transparent pockets to support the work process. To have all items in view in the correct order that functions at the same time as a checklist. It also offers resilience in case of skipped process steps because the skipped item is still visible and ready for a deferred use if apt. This functionality corresponds to the design principle of affordance, that is, the information contained in an object's physical appearance to how it can/should be used, originally introduced by Gibson (2014). In a controlled trial, this approach turned out to be associated with a lower rate of line infections. They also performed an economic analysis (Nelson et al. 2015). Clack et al. (2019) gave a detailed account of an iterative user-centred design approach to isolation room signage. The influence of unconscious human factors

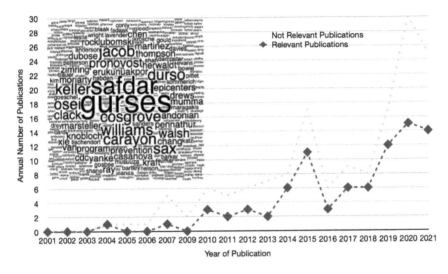

FIGURE 10.3 Number of publications on human factors in infection prevention (PubMed Search)

Legend for Figure 10.3 Literature search in PubMed using search strategies through PubMed search with "(human factors[Title/Abstract]) AND (infection prevention)" on 31 December 2021 and hand selected into "Relevant Publications" and "Not Relevant Publications." Relevant was defined as concerning both human factors engineering and infection prevention, even if either was not the main topic of the publication. The inserted word cloud lists all authors in "Relevant Publications," the size of the name representing the number of appearances.

was investigated by Birnbach et al. (2013) who found that lemon scent present in the environment increased hand hygiene adherence against a control group in a simulation setting. The same group investigated the influence of pictures of eyes versus flowers attached to handrub dispensers on hand hygiene behaviour (King et al. 2016).

Personal protective equipment (PPE) was a frequent topic for HF/E. Salehi et al. (2018) found 13 design improvement opportunities in PPE in the literature and through observations. The Ebola threat motivated an HF/E evaluation of the infectious risks associated with PPE doffing (Gurses et al. 2019). More recently, the SARS-CoV-2 pandemic that started in 2020 brought more HF/E expertise to IPC. Carayon and Perry (2020) suggested the SEIPS framework as a usable lens to manage real-time work system adaptation as the pandemic evolved. An example of such practise is reported by Fadaak et al. (2021). An inter-disciplinary team of HF/E, ethnography, and IPC experts assisted the conversion of a surgical ward into a COVID-19 unit. They used walkthroughs, simulations, and ethnography to identify important safety gaps in care delivery processes. Keller et al. mapped results of observations and interviews regarding physical distancing in the hospital onto the SEIPS work system components and identified barriers, facilitators, and healthcare provider-suggested solutions (Keller et al. 2021). A typical HF/E finding was the influence of unsuitable infrastructure that led people to being too close. Even if the redesign of lookalike/sound-alike syringes can seem low hanging fruit, it might fail due to complexity at the organisational level (Clack, Kuster et al. 2014).

10.7 THE EXAMPLE OF HAND HYGIENE

Nothing in IPC exemplifies the policy-behaviour gap more than hand hygiene. It lends itself therefore to evaluate the potential benefit of an HF/E approach to IPC. Among the very early applications of an explicit HF/E approach to an IPC problem was the WHO "My five moments of hand hygiene" concept that considered mental models and was created through iterative prototyping and bedside simulations (Sax et al. 2007, 2009). It found a global diffusion through the promotion by WHO within a multifaceted implementation framework, named the "five avenues of action" (WHO 2009), and has led to an increase in patient safety worldwide (Allegranzi et al. 2013).

Any HF/E approach to the problem, in this case hand hygiene, would start with a "first principal" analysis. There is good evidence that hands touch surfaces frequently and constantly (Clack, Scotoni et al. 2017) and transport pathogens from one surface to another (Longtin et al. 2014; Wolfensberger et al. 2018; Boyce et al. 2021). The risk for cross-contamination and infection has been established through observations and expert evaluation resulting in an actionable risk framework (Clack, Schmutz et al. 2014, Clack, Passerini et al. 2018). It therefore makes sense to interrupt this transmission chain, as suggested by the "My five moments of hand hygiene" concept. There are, however, several points to be considered. First, there is also convincing evidence that most of this transfer of microorganisms is not harmful. Exchange of microbiota among household members happens constantly without harm. The same is probably true for healthcare settings. Studies with surrogate tracers show how quickly and far microorganisms spread (Oelberg et al. 2000; Ullrich et al. 2022). This high rate of transfer does not match the much lower occurrence of HAI. Moreover, the pathophysiology of most HAI speaks against exogenous routes of infection. Catheter-associated urinary tract infections (CAUTI), for example, are much more likely due to endogenous transmission of gut flora from the perianal region to the (catheterised) urinary tract (Jacobsen et al. 2008). In consequence, hand hygiene would do little to prevent CAUTI—if it is not during catheter insertion. Second, the moment of a relevant transmission (risk) remains hidden to human senses.

According to this reasoning, an artificial system would be useful if it alerted HCP of the presence of a situation of high risk of a "harmful" transmission and then pointed to show the preventive effect of hand hygiene. The alert would be timely, emotionally engaging and non-disturbing, and hand hygiene would be made easy and pleasurable. We could imagine this system to receive inputs from multiple sensors, patient records, HCP personal behaviour patterns, location and real-time microbiology data to identify moments with higher risk density. We could further make the pathogens "visible" to HCPs. However, the "irony of automatization" must be considered, the fact that the attempt to solve a problem by automatization can backfire and make the system even more complex (Shorrock & Williams 2016).

Meanwhile, we must perform hand hygiene 1,000 times or more to prevent one harmful transmission. In this situation, an HF/E approach could help to over-represent the risk and minimise the "cost" for hand hygiene. Table 10.1 provides a "silent brainstorming" relating human factors to potential HF/E design solutions. Of course, such rough ideas would have to be further evaluated, selected, prototyped and tested.

TABLE 10.1   The author's "silent brainstorming" on human factors and potential human factors engineering solutions for hand hygiene in health care [752]

HUMAN FACTORS	POTENTIAL HF/E SOLUTIONS
Risk perception Humans react to immediate experience of risk. However, microorganisms are invisible, and infections manifest themselves with latency. There is no immediate reaction when hand hygiene is not done. Cumulative statistical risk is not easily perceived and translated in the current situation. The perception of the outcome of one's behaviour is of the three dimensions of the theory of planned behaviour.	(Electronic) monitoring and immediate feedback at the point of care (auditive, haptic, visual, etc.) displaying each patient's cumulative number of times touched by unclean hands. Feedback of each HCP's "transmission footprint." Display of the overall hand transmission risk at each moment considering all hand hygiene opportunities in the hospital. Real-time and world use of surrogate tracers that show transmission pathway. Repetitive exposure to virtual reality scenarios and serious games to maintain mental models of transmission. Redesign of hand hygiene moments to better consider the sweet spot between human intrinsic motivation and microbiological effect.
Habits Humans form habits and "muscle memory," which helps to execute tasks automatically. Such behaviours can be triggered through perceived cues without cognitive load.	Conditioning training that are triggered by cues to action (consistent with natural care environment) to build a habit ("clicker training"). Consistent appearance (form, colour) and location of handrub dispensers. Rewarding sound or light feedback to handrub use to reinforce habit. These must be nonintrusive, for example, only intermittently.
Mental models Humans make sense of the environment through mental models. Mental models can be different between HCPs, which can lead to perceived different patient zone limitations (Bogdanovic et al. 2019) and, thus, transmission risk (Sax & Clack 2015).	Patient zone marking, for example, zones with different surface colours (better than just lines that show borders). Spacious room structure with clear grouping of surfaces that belong to the same (patient) zone. Critical sites markings on patients, for example, small hand symbols/colour markings on invasive sites that require prior hand hygiene. Sensors with sound or haptic signal when approaching critical site; random intermittent occurrence to avoid alert fatigue. Mindfulness practice to internalise HH as important moments in patient care. Training HCPs in observing one's own mental models. Training HCPs adopting a system view and seeing opportunities for system improvements.
Attention The moment of approaching a patient or the moment just before executing an aseptic task are usually moments of high cognitive load. In such moments, there is no capacity for conscious decision-making.	Workflow-optimised handrub dispenser location. High signal-to-noise ratio for handrub dispenser design against background. See also "Habit" and "Movement detection."

(Continued)

TABLE 10.1 (Continued)

HUMAN FACTORS	POTENTIAL HF/E SOLUTIONS
Visual movement detection The periphery of the retina contains rods, which is associated with increased movement detection (and low light sensitivity but lack of colour detection).	Handrub dispenser design with moving elements that are activated when a person comes closer.
Social norms, culture Humans are "social animals." The perception of what others think of them is one of the three dimensions of the theory of planned behaviour. Culture ("how things are done here") is very stable and has therefore been called "social DNA."	Signs with social norm activation, for example, picture of eyes [55] thank-you message from patients and family. Framing of feedback reports as social norm. Establish a positive culture of HH through consistent role modelling by important personalities for distinct healthcare provider groups.
Sensory pleasure, "flow" Humans take pleasure in certain sensory experiences, rhythms, and movements, often experienced as "flow." The notion of something taking too much time can in reality be an awkward break of the flow.	Convenient position of handrub dispensers for flow of movement and natural location at indicated moment, for example, beginning of walkway into room to give 15″ for hand rubbing, no awkward turning or bending to reach the dispenser. Pleasurable haptics of handrub dispenser activation and handrub product. Space to deposit carried objects to free hands for HH. Workflow design to avoid task competition and ambiguities about priorities.
Behavioural control Humans like to feel in control of things. The perception of how likely one can perform an action is one of the three dimensions of the theory of planned behaviour.	Clear, simple rules that match actual work environment and flow, even at the compromise of a 100% microbiological security. Handrub dispenser delivers product reliably and without any delay upon activation. Touchless delivery of handrub.
Instincts, associations Primary instincts, for example, self-preservation, empathy, disgust.	"Priming" room scent, handrub product scent [55]. Surface structure or visual aspect to induce disgust and motivate to clean hands.

10.8 HF/E-AS-DONE VERSUS HF/E-AS-IMAGINED

Over the last 15 years, HF/E has been recognised by the IPC community as an opportunity, but its implementation in IPC teams does not seem to have matched its praise. Why is this so? Storr et al. (2013) recognise the lack of resources and call for an increased capacity and capability of HF/E principles in IPC. Similarly, Patel and Kallen (2018) highlighted the fact that HF/E in IPC is resource intensive and that HF/E expertise is lacking in most if not all hospitals. They state,

> Ultimately, the value of human factors approaches to infection prevention will depend on the ability not only to just identify and describe challenges to best practice but also to successfully overcome challenges through effective interventions that improve adherence and reduce HAIs.

It is hard to define what good HF/E in IPC should look like, especially because it overlaps with neighbouring efforts to bring scientific discovery to the bedside (Figure 10.4). Nevertheless, in my view the following requirements apply.

First, HF/E must take a holistic systems approach and evolve with our increasing understanding of how to best consider adaptive complexity (Hollnagel 2014). Humans find solutions in contradictory and ill-defined situations, which must be anticipated in the design process and appreciated as a resource (Turner & Baker 2020). Furthermore, IPC must be seen within the optimisation of the overall objective of health care, its main "product," sustainable improvement of the health of patients.

Second, HF/E in IPC cannot be seen independent of overall scientific progress, especially our understanding of the nature of infections. This is well exemplified by the increasing knowledge of SARS-CoV-2 transmission pathways with its immediate relevance to prevention measures and policy. Only better knowledge of the invisible world of infections will help us to upgrade architecture, devices, processes and mental models. The application of artificial intelligence to IPC will accelerate this knowledge (Fitzpatrick et al. 2020). The

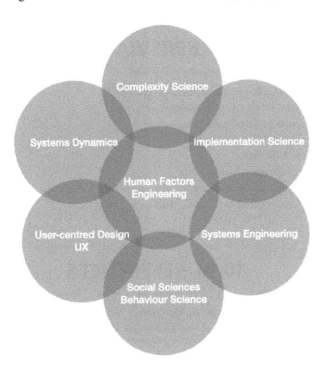

FIGURE 10.4 Knowledge fields overlapping with human factors engineering

introduction of AI, robotics and new real-time diagnostics in health care will also force us to rethink the distribution of work between humans and artificial systems. This will lead to new challenges for interface design and updates in HF/E regarding mental models. Moreover, if we eventually succeed in modifying the work environment very effectively with the help of advanced (AI-aided) HF/E design approach, an ethical and technical challenge arises. What if we fall short of understanding the true dynamics of infectious risks in health care and, hence, guide HCPs in the wrong direction? This question became very concrete when we were working on a virtual reality hand hygiene trainer in which we had to decide on the exact behaviour of the visible microorganisms (Clack, Hirt et al. 2018).

Third, HF/E must remain first and foremost an engineering discipline. While the first step is to recognise and appreciate the principles of HF/E, this is not enough. Solid education and practical experience with the application of HF/E principles in the harsh reality of health care is crucial (Catchpole et al. 2020). Only professionals with experience and arguments, for example, can make a difference on the "battlefield" of competing interests in planning a new hospital building. Furthermore, the HF/E toolset must co-evolve within health care between traditional HF/E tools and new inventions. How to best integrate this practical expertise in IPC and hospitals could be a formidable macro-ergonomic HF/E challenge on its own. It will also involve creating specific educational opportunities, for example, MD-PhD tracks in HF/E and IPC, but also educating HCP in systems thinking.

Today, I view the idea and expertise of HF/E as a gravitational centre that holds great promise for IPC, but as the ubiquitous persistence of flawed design in everyday life shows, there is still a long way to go.

10.9 ABBREVIATIONS

CAUTI   Catheter-associated urinary tract infections
FDA   US Food and Drug and Administration
HAI   Healthcare-associated infections
HF/E   Human factors and ergonomics
HCP   Healthcare provider
IPC   Infection prevention and control
PPE   Personal protective equipment
SEIPS   Systems Engineering Initiative for Patient Safety

10.10 REFERENCES

Allegranzi B, Gayet-Ageron A, Damani N, Bengaly L, McLaws M-L, Moro M-L, et al. Global implementation of WHO's multimodal strategy for improvement of hand hygiene: A quasi-experimental study. *The Lancet Infectious Diseases*. 2013;13:843–51.
Altman M, Huang TTK, Breland JY. Design thinking in health care. *Preventing Chronic Disease*. 2018;15:E117.

Anderson J, Gosbee LL, Bessesen M, Williams L. Using human factors engineering to improve the effectiveness of infection prevention and control. *Critical Care Medicine* [Internet]. 2010;38:S269–81. Available from: http://meta.wkhealth.com/pt/pt-core/template-journal/lwwgateway/media/landingpage.htm?issn=0090-3493&volume=38&issue=8&spage=S269

Anil S. Preface: The brain as a prediction machine. In: ["Mendonça, Dina", "Curado, Manuel", "Gouveia, S."] Steven, editors. *The Philosophy and Science of Predictive Processing* [Internet]. 1st ed. London: Bloomsbury Academic; 2020. pp. xiv–xvii. Available from: www.bloomsburycollections.com/book/the-philosophy-and-science-of-predictive-processing/preface-the-brain-as-a-prediction-machine/

Baumgart A, Neuhauser D. Frank and Lillian Gilbreth: Scientific management in the operating room. *Quality and Safety in Health Care*. 2009;18:413–5.

Birnbach DJ, King D, Vlaev I, Rosen LF, Harvey PD. Impact of environmental olfactory cues on hand hygiene behaviour in a simulated hospital environment: A randomized study. *Journal of Hospital Infection*. 2013;85:79–81.

Bogdanovic J, Petralito S, Passerini S, Sax H, Manser T, Clack L. Exploring healthcare providers' mental models of the infection prevention "patient zone"—a concept mapping study. *Antimicrobial Resistance and Infection Control*. 2019;8:138.

Boyce JM, Havill NL, Guercia KA, Moore BA. Microbial burden on environmental surfaces in patient rooms before daily cleaning—Analysis of multiple confounding variables. *Infection Control Hospital Epidemiology*. 2021;1–5.

Branaghan RJ, O'Brian JS, Hildebrand EA, Foster LB. Humanizing healthcare—human factors for medical device design. *Springer*. 2021:159–83.

Browne RC, Darcus HD, Roberts CG, Conrad R, Edholm OG, Hick WE, et al. Ergonomics Research Society. *BMJ*. 1950;1:1009–1009.

Cafazzo JA, St-Cyr O. From discovery to design: The evolution of human factors in healthcare. *Healthcare Quarterly (Toronto, Ont)*. 2012;15 Spec No:24–9.

Carayon P. *Handbook of Human Factors and Ergonomics in Health Care and Patient Safety*. 2nd ed. Carayon P, editor. Boca Raton, FL: CRC Press; 2011.

Carayon P, Hundt AS, Karsh B-T, Gurses AP, Alvarado CJ, Smith M, et al. Work system design for patient safety: The SEIPS model. *Quality and Safety in Health Care*. 2006;15 Suppl 1:i50–8.

Carayon P, Karsh B-T, Gurses AP, Holden RJ, Hoonakker P, Hundt AS, et al. Macroergonomics in health care quality and patient safety. *Reviews of Human Factors and Ergonomics*. 2013;8:4–54.

Carayon P, Perry S. Human factors and ergonomics systems approach to the COVID-19 healthcare crisis. *International Journal for Quality in Health Care*. 2020;33:mzaa109.

Carayon P, Wooldridge A, Hoonakker P, Hundt AS, Kelly MM. SEIPS 3.0: Human-centered design of the patient journey for patient safety. *Applied Ergonomics*. 2020;84:103033.

Catchpole K, Bowie P, Fouquet S, Rivera J, Hignett S. Frontiers in human factors: Embedding specialists in multi-disciplinary efforts to improve healthcare. *International Journal for Quality in Health Care*. 2020;33:13–8.

Chabris C, Simons D. *The Invisible Gorilla*. New York, NY: Crown Archetype; 2010.

Chaparro A, Keebler JR, Lazzara EH, Diamond A. Checklists: A review of their origins, benefits, and current uses as a cognitive aid in medicine. *Ergonomics DESQ Human Factors Applied*. 2019;27:21–6.

Clack L, Hirt C, Wenger M, Saleschus D, Kunz A, Sax H. VIRTUE—A Virtual reality trainer for hand hygiene. *2018 9th International Conference on Information, Intelligence, Systems Applied IISA*. 2018;00:1–2.

Clack L, Kuster SP, Giger H, Giuliani F, Sax H. Low-hanging fruit for human factors design in infection prevention-still too high to reach? *American Journal of Infection Control* [Internet]. 2014a;42:679–81. Available from: http://secure.jbs.elsevierhealth.com/action/cookieAbsent

Clack L, Passerini S, Wolfensberger A, Sax H, Manser T. Frequency and nature of infectious risk moments during acute care based on the INFORM structured classification taxonomy. *Infection Control & Hospital Epidemiology*. 2018;39:272–9.

Clack L, Sax H. Annals for hospitalists inpatient notes—human factors engineering and inpatient care—new ways to solve old problems. *Annals of Internal Medicine*. 2017;166:HO2.

Clack L, Schmutz J, Manser T, Sax H. Infectious risk moments: A novel, human factors-informed approach to infection prevention. *Infection Control Hospital Epidemiology*. 2014b;35:1051–5.

Clack L, Scotoni M, Wolfensberger A, Sax H. "First-person view" of pathogen transmission and hand hygiene—use of a new head-mounted video capture and coding tool. *Antimicrobial Resistance and Infection Control*. 2017;6;108.

Clack L, Stühlinger M, Meier M-T, Wolfensberger A, Sax H. User-centred participatory design of visual cues for isolation precautions. *Antimicrobial Resistance Information*. 2019;8;179.

Donabedian A. *The Quality of Medical Care. Science* (New York, NY). 1978;200:856–64.

Drews FA, Bakdash JZ, Gleed JR. Improving central line maintenance to reduce central line-associated bloodstream infections. *American Journal of Infection Control*. 2017;45:1224–30.

Drews FA, Visnovsky LC, Mayer J. Human factors engineering contributions to infection prevention and control. *Human Factors*. 2019;61:693–701.

Fadaak R, Davies JM, Blaak MJ, Conly J, Haslock J, Kenny A, et al. Rapid conversion of an in-patient hospital unit to accommodate COVID-19: An interdisciplinary human factors, ethnography, and infection prevention and control approach. *PLoS One*. 2021;16:e0245212.

Fitzpatrick F, Doherty A, Lacey G. Using artificial intelligence in infection prevention. *Current Treatment Options in Infectious Diseases*. 2020;12:135–44.

Gibson JJ. *The Ecological Approach to Visual Perception*. New York, NY: Psychology Press Classic Edition; 2014.

Gurses AP, Dietz AS, Nowakowski E, Andonian J, Schiffhauer M, Billman C, et al. Human factors-based risk analysis to improve the safety of doffing enhanced personal protective equipment. *Infect Control Hosp Epidemiology*. 2019;40:178–86.

Holden RJ, Carayon P, Gurses AP, Hoonakker P, Hundt AS, Ozok AA, et al. SEIPS 2.0: A human factors framework for studying and improving the work of healthcare professionals and patients. *Ergonomics*. 2013;56:1669–86.

Hollnagel E. Human factors/ergonomics as a systems discipline? "The human use of human beings" revisited. *Applied Ergonomics*. 2014;45:40–4.

Hollnagel E. The nitty gritty of human factors. In: Shorrock S and Williams C, editor. *Human Factors and Ergonomics in Practice*. Boca Raton, FL: Taylor & Francis; 2017:45–64.

Human Factors and Ergonomics Society [Internet]. [cited 2021 Dec 18]. Available from: www.hfes.org

Human Factors and Ergonomics Society Definition [Internet]. [cited 2021 Dec 18]. Available from: www.hfes.org/About-HFES/What-is-Human-Factors-and-Ergonomics#professional_societies

Iedema R, Hor S-Y, Wyer M, et al. An innovative approach to strengthening health professionals' infection control and limiting hospital-acquired infection: Video-reflexive ethnography. *BMJ Innovations*. 2015;1:157–62.

International Ergonomics Society [Internet]. Available from: https://iea.cc

Jacob JT, Herwaldt LA, Durso FT, Program CPE. Preventing healthcare-associated infections through human factors engineering. *Current Treatment Options in Infectious Diseases*. 2018;31:353–8.

Jacobsen SM, Stickler DJ, Mobley HLT, Shirtliff ME. Complicated catheter-associated urinary tract infections due to escherichia coli and proteus mirabilis. *Clinical Microbiology Reviews*. 2008;21:26–59.

Jastrzebowski W. *Outline of Ergonomics, or the science of Work Based Upon Truths Drawn from Science of Nature 1857*. Warszawa, PL: Central Institute for Labour Protection; 2000.

Johnson-Laird PN. *Mental Models*. Cambridge, MA: Harvard University Press; 1983.

Johnson-Laird PN. *How We Reason*. Oxford: Oxford University Press; 2006.

Karwowski W. The discipline of human factors and ergonomics. In: Salvendy G, editor. *Handbook of Human Factors and Ergonomics [Internet]*. Hoboken, NJ: John Wiley & Sons; 2021. Available from: https://onlinelibrary.wiley.com/doi/book/10.1002/9781118131350

Keller SC, Salinas AB, Oladapo-Shittu O, Cosgrove SE, Lewis-Cherry R, Vecchio-Pagan B, et al. Barriers to physical distancing among healthcare workers on an academic hospital unit during the coronavirus disease 2019 (COVID-19) pandemic. *Infection Control & Hospital Epidemiology*. 2021;1–7.

King D, Vlaev I, Everett-Thomas R, Fitzpatrick M, Darzi A, Birnbach DJ. "Priming" hand hygiene compliance in clinical environments. *Health Psychology: Official Journal of the Division of Health Psychology, American Psychological Association*. 2016;35:96–101.

KLM-PAA. Joint Report [Internet]. 1978 Dec. Available from: www.project-tenerife.com/engels/PDF/Tenerife.pdf

Kohn LT. To err is human: An interview with the institute of medicine's Linda Kohn. *Joint Commission Journal on Quality Improvement*. 2000;26:227–34.

Kohn LT, Corrigan Janet M, Donaldson MS, editors. *To Err is Human: Building a Safer Health System* [Internet]. National Academy Press; 2000. Available from: http://books.google.com/books?id=1NSGBPzemrYC&printsec=frontcover

Longtin Y, Schneider A, Tschopp C, Renzi G, Gayet-Ageron A, Schrenzel J, et al. Contamination of stethoscopes and physicians' hands after a physical examination. *Mayo Clinic Proceedings Mayo Clinic*. 2014;89:291–9.

Meister D. *The History of Human Factors and Ergonomics*. Boca Raton, FL: CRC Press; 2018:33–88.

Mental Models Global Laboratory [Internet]. [cited 2021 Dec 5]. Available from: www.modeltheory.org

Mouloua SA, Ball RV, Ferraro JC, Mouloua M. The history of human factors in healthcare: From its emergence 50 years ago to COVID-19. *Proceedings International Symposium on Human Factors and Ergonomics in Health Care*. 2021;10:165–9.

Nelson RE, Angelovic AW, Nelson SD, Gleed JR, Drews FA. An economic analysis of adherence engineering to improve use of best practices during central line maintenance procedures. *Infect Control Hosp Epidemiology*. 2015;36:550–6.

Norris B, West J, Anderson O, Davey G, Brodie A. Taking ergonomics to the bedside-a multi-disciplinary approach to designing safer healthcare. *Applied Ergonomics*. 2013;45:629–38.

Oelberg DG, Joyner SE, Jiang X, Laborde D, Islam MP, Pickering LK. Detection of pathogen transmission in neonatal nurseries using DNA markers as surrogate indicators. *Pediatrics*. 2000;105:311–5.

Patel PR, Kallen AJ. Human factors and systems engineering: The future of infection prevention? *Infect Control Hosp Epidemiology*. 2018;39:849–51.

Pennathur PR, Herwaldt LA. Role of human factors engineering in infection prevention: Gaps and opportunities. *Current Treatment Options in Infectious Diseases*. 2017;9:230–49.

Plsek PE, Greenhalgh T. Complexity science: The challenge of complexity in health care. *BMJ Innovations*. 2001;323:625–8.

Salehi H, Pennathur PR, Silva JPD, Herwaldt LA. Examining health care personal protective equipment use through a human factors engineering and product design lens. *American Journal of Infection Control*. 2018;47:595–8.

Sax H, Allegranzi B, Chraïti M-N, Boyce J, Larson E, Pittet D. The World Health Organization hand hygiene observation method. *American Journal of Infection Control*. 2009;37:827–34.

Sax H, Allegranzi B, Uçkay I, Larson E, Boyce J, Pittet D. "My five moments for hand hygiene": A user-centred design approach to understand, train, monitor and report hand hygiene. *Journal of Hospital Infection*. 2007;67:9–21.

Sax H, Clack L. Mental models: A basic concept for human factors design in infection prevention. *Journal of Hospital Infection*. 2015;89:335–9.

Schmutz J, Eppich WJ, Hoffmann F, Heimberg E, Manser T. Five steps to develop checklists for evaluating clinical performance: An integrative approach. *Academic Medicine: Journal of the Association of American Medical Colleges*. 2014;89:996–1005.

Schreiber PW, Sax H, Wolfensberger A, Clack L, Kuster SP, Swissnoso. The preventable proportion of healthcare-associated infections 2005–2016: Systematic review and meta-analysis. *Infection Control & Hospital Epidemiology*. 2018;34:1–19.

Shorrock S, Williams C. *Human Factors and Ergonomics in Practice*. New York: Routledge; 2016.

Staiger TO. *The Value of Systems and Complexity Sciences for Healthcare*. Berlin: Springer Publishers; 2016:69–78.

Stanton NA. Special issue on human factors and ergonomics methods. *Human Factors and Ergonomics in Manufacturing*. 2022;32:3–5.

Stanton NA, Salmon PM, Rafferty LA, Walker GH, Barber C, Jenkins DP. *Human Factor Methods: A Practical Guide for Engineering and Design*. London: CRC Press; 2013.

Storr J, Wigglesworth N, Kilpatrick C. *Integrating Human Factors with Infection Prevention and Control*. London: Health Foundation; 2013.

Turner JR, Baker R. Just doing the do: A case study testing creativity and innovative processes as complex adaptive systems. *New Horizons in Adult Education and Human Resource Development*. 2020;32:40–61.

U.S. Department of Health and Human Services, Food and Drug Administration. *Applying Human Factors and Usability Engineering to Medical Devices: Guidance for Industry and Food and Drug Administration Staff* [Internet]. U.S. Department of Health and Human Services, Food and Drug Administration; 2016 Feb. Available from: www.fda.gov/media/80481/download

Ullrich C, Luescher AM, Koch J, Grass RN, Sax H. Silica nanoparticles with encapsulated DNA (SPED) to trace the spread of pathogens in healthcare. *Antimicrobial Resistance and Infection Control*. 2022;11:4. https://doi.org/10.1186/s13756-021-01041-3

Vicente KJ. *Cognitive Work Analysis*. New York: CRC Press; 1999.

Vicente KJ. *The Human Factor* [Internet]. Psychology Press; 2004. Available from: http://books.google.com/books?id=TSW11Tc4arIC&dq=intitle:the+human+factor+inauthor:vicente&hl=&cd=1&source=gbs_api

Walton M, Woodward H, Staalduinen SV, Lemer C, Greaves F, Noble D, et al. The WHO patient safety curriculum guide for medical schools. *Quality and Safety in Health Care*. 2010;19:542–6.

WHO. *Save Lives: Clean Your Hand. Guide to Implementation. A Guide to the Implementation of the WHO Multimodal Hand Hygiene Improvement Strategy* [Internet]. World Health Organization; 2009. Available from: http://whqlibdoc.who.int/hq/2009/WHO_IER_PSP_2009.02_eng.pdf

Wolfensberger A, Clack L, Kuster SP, Passerini S, Mody L, Chopra V, et al. Transfer of pathogens to and from patients, healthcare providers, and medical devices during care activity-a systematic review and meta-analysis. *Infection Control Hospital Epidemiology*. 2018;39:1–15.

Xie A, Carayon P. A systematic review of human factors and ergonomics (HFE)-based healthcare system redesign for quality of care and patient safety. *Ergonomics*. 2015;58:33–49.

How We Talk About Infection Prevention and Hand Hygiene Matters for Behaviour Change

11

Claire Kilpatrick and Julie Storr

Contents

> Words can be like X-rays if you use them properly—they'll go through anything.
>
> (Huxley 2007) Aldous Huxley, *Brave New World*

11.1 INTRODUCTION TO THE ISSUE

There are numerous examples of the influence of words on behaviour. From the overt propaganda employed by Winston Churchill during World War II (Crespo-Fernández 2013)

DOI: 10.1201/9781003379393-14

to the application of neuro linguistic programming (NLP) as a marketing tool (Skinner and Stephens 2003). Churchill's resorted to emotive, intemperate and violent language as a mass persuasion device to attack enemies, akin to a loaded weapon. Similar approaches, including using the language of fear as a public health strategy, have been seen during the COVID-19 pandemic (Stolow et al. 2020). Studies over many decades have highlighted the importance of communication and language for public health as well as between healthcare providers and patients.

Social marketing, which aims to address behaviour change by combining communications and products that can enhance health and wellbeing, has been recognised in the field of infection prevention for some time. Storr and Sax writing in one of the only books focused solely on hand hygiene for medical professionals (Storr and Sax 2017) noted the importance of engaging social science experts if future gains are to be made and the necessary influence on healthcare worker behaviour to be achieved. To put this in context with regards to improvement efforts, social marketing falls into the fourth element of what WHO terms a multimodal improvement strategy (MMIS) (WHO 2009), namely, the importance of addressing reminders and communications in infection prevention programmes.

But as noted, words, as part of communication and marketing efforts, carry power. Over 20 years ago Kretzer and Larson (1998) challenged the use of the word "compliance" in an infection prevention and control (IPC) context and suggested alternatives. However, Coles' more recent study (Cole 2014) highlighted the continued disproportionate use of the word in policies, compared to alternatives.

11.2 A UNIVERSAL ISSUE

Against this context and appreciating that hand hygiene in health care is often perceived as a basic intervention, or even "common sense" (Jumaa 2005), the authors of this chapter embarked on a piece of work to delve deeper into the issue. An exploratory language exercise was undertaken across 24 discrete focus groups in seven countries. Participants were selected using a convenience approach with participants invited to share their perceptions of words commonly used in association with hand hygiene improvement. This included talking to infection preventionists, nurses, doctors, senior management and a diverse range of other health workers and managers. This novel exercise (Kilpatrick and Storr 2017) aimed to stimulate the infection prevention and academic communities to revisit the words used within policies/guidelines and day-to-day communications in their quest to bring about the socially desired change [hand hygiene at the right time]. It was also seen as an opportunity to provide a powerful motivator towards enhancing training and education and monitoring and evaluation activities; both of which form some of the remaining elements of the MMIS. The results of this exercise will be returned to later in the chapter.

11.3 WHY IS BEHAVIOUR CHANGE IMPORTANT IN INFECTION PREVENTION, AND HOW DOES COMMUNICATION RELATE TO BEHAVIOUR CHANGE?

Addressing behaviour change in relation to hand hygiene and overall IPC has in essence been notable across the literature for the last decades. In 2012, Huis et al. explored the content and effectiveness of a range of strategies to improve hand hygiene adherence using a detailed coding taxonomy of behaviour change techniques targeting major behavioural determinants (Huis et al. 2012). This work sheds interesting light on frequently used improvement strategies and how they work. Their findings reinforced that combinations of different determinants yield better results, suggesting a need for more creativity in the application of improvement activities whilst acknowledging WHO's MMIS approach. Addressing the use of words or language within reminders and communications, as one part of IPC programme improvement efforts, could be linked to the notion of more "creative application." In a similar vein to Huis et al., Edwards et al. (2012) presented their systematic review on optimising infection prevention by use of behaviour change. This was an important reinforcement on the need for behaviour change consideration within this context. Importantly, it outlined that there had been investment in behaviour change strategies but minimal evaluation. The authors noted that only two identified studies contained social marketing, which encompasses reminders and communications.

Within the WHO hand hygiene guidelines (WHO 2009) there is a chapter dedicated to behavioural considerations, which highlights that human behaviours are a function of people's perceptions and as such are influenced by multiple factors, including culture, environment, education and, in part, communications. McLaws and Sax (2017), in their chapter on behaviour and hand hygiene, also explored the fact that health worker behaviours span professionalism and altruism and described the role of social marketing models in relation to the perceived needs of an audience in order to address the perceived benefits to an idea, hand hygiene. The WHO annual hand hygiene campaign held each 5 May is a way in which the need for hand hygiene improvement is regularly marketed or communicated in order to ensure an ongoing global profile (WHO SAVE LIVES—Clean Your Hands 2022). Slogans and calls to action are employed each year, aimed at the primary audience, those working within health care. However, aside from translating the messages into the official United Nation languages, which involves considering user interpretation to some extent, there is no evidence that the language used is tested on the recipients of the messages. The slogans and calls to action are however formulated by communications as well as technical experts. In the associated WHO hand hygiene improvement tools released each 5 May, medical, or so-called "technical," language tends to predominate, and the word *compliance* is featured.

An evaluation of the national cleanyourhands campaign™ in England, which included a range of communication strategies (Stone et al. 2012), demonstrated an associated impact on hand hygiene adherence and suggested this MMIS had an important role in reducing rates of some healthcare associated infections. The evaluation team included one of the behavioural psychologists who subsequently went on to codevelop the ground-breaking Behaviour Change Wheel (Michie et al. 2011) and associated COM-B (capability, opportunity, motivation—behaviour) approach. In an interview with Michie (2013), she highlights that the cleanyourhands campaign™ can be conceptualised in terms of capability, opportunity and motivation, describing how it addressed motivation by engaging hospitals in creating and displaying motivational posters in the wards, regularly changed to prevent habituation to them. The behaviour change wheel was further presented to an IPC audience through a publication in 2016, which outlined the framework in order to guide behaviour change intervention design (Atkins 2016) and has also been the focus of a scoping review by the University of the West of London outlined in 2021 (Greene and Wilson 2021).

Finally, communication, and the use of words, has also been raised within the field of antimicrobial resistance (AMR), highlighting that language in the context of behaviour change is of growing concern in associated fields. In an article in *Nature*, Mendelson et al. in (2017) raised the point that a failure to use words clearly means compromising the global response to AMR. The authors highlighted the unfamiliarity of terms and interchangeable use of terms as key issues, outlining that all have the potential to be counterproductive and lead to lack of engagement as people feel powerless to do anything. Mendelson et al. draw parallels with other high-profile topics such as climate change and HIV/AIDS. Subsequently, the Wellcome Trust in the UK published a report on "Reframing resistance; how to communicate about antimicrobial resistance effectively" outlining five principles for framing AMR messages and language to encourage action (Wellcome Trust 2019).

11.4 WHAT DO WE KNOW NOW ABOUT THE LANGUAGE OF HAND HYGIENE?

Etymology is defined in *The New Oxford English Dictionary* (2001) as the study of the origin of words and their meaning over time. If one were to categorise the etymology of hand hygiene across the late twentieth and early twenty-first centuries, there would be broad agreement that it falls within the medical model of health. There is a standardised language that has been adopted almost universally. The conceptual basis for this lies in the world of microbiology and medicine with its emphasis on Latinate or old English terms and words and, to some extent in more latter years, quality improvement language. The WHO Guidelines on hand hygiene in health care (WHO 2009) reflect this, alongside almost every other guideline produced by national organizations, academia and individual healthcare institutions. Whilst there is currently no official taxonomy of hand hygiene, there exists an accepted way of talking about it that seems to display little variation.

Outside of hand hygiene in health care, attention has been paid to language and the feelings evoked. Curtis, a public health expert and world leader in the field of hygiene as a method of stopping diarrhoeal illnesses in children in low- and middle-income countries is a case in point. She consistently highlighted that the feeling of disgust is common in all humans and a prototypical emotion, evoking feelings such as "stop, don't touch" and that this feeling evolved in our ancestors to avoid infectious diseases (Curtis 2011). Curtis frequently asked listeners and readers to think of other people's body fluids, pustules, using toilet brushes to clean dishes and generally used key, everyday emotive words in her efforts to influence behaviour.

Although not the focus of this chapter, it is hard to overlook the language used in the context of hand hygiene improvement efforts within the COVID-19 pandemic. Early in the pandemic in the UK, politicians and public health professionals attempted to promote hand hygiene through the use of the song "Happy Birthday," focusing on the time required to perform the action of hand hygiene (The Telegraph 2020). This was an interesting choice and one which Kilpatrick questioned in an opinion piece, noting that while the song perhaps made for a good 20 seconds of television, its association with celebration and light-heartedness could be considered infantile (Kilpatrick 2021). The intention was no doubt admirable. and it could be argued that every little helps. However the issue is that words and associations matter, and we should be open to probing and critiquing the language of IPC. Nevertheless, many common words are used in the quest for hand hygiene improvement. In 2012, personal conversations by the authors with a speechwriter, presentation specialist and blogger on language and communication highlighted the need for more focus and creativity in the language employed by IPC professionals to strengthen behaviour change efforts. To illustrate the power of words and their influence on behaviours, a story about a fish was shared! The pilchard, a small fish from the herring family, was a staple part of the UK diet during and immediately after the Second World War. As the years passed by, sales declined, and the pilchard went out of fashion, being associated in the mind of the public with wartime rationing and a time that people wanted to forget. As the story goes, a local businessman in the UK county of Cornwall decided it was time for a rebrand. In a bid to change the public perception, he changed the name, from pilchard to Cornish sardines. This simple decision to change a word resulted in a massive change in perception that manifested in increased sales and a renaissance in the consumption of this tiny fish. Changing a word can, it appears, change behaviours (Simpson 2021).

The subsequent exploratory exercise, conducted over 2013 and 2014 (Kilpatrick and Storr 2017), aimed to address the barriers and facilitators that influence human behaviour and the influence of prevalent language on whether hand hygiene occurs at the correct moments. The approach involved a rapid review of the literature to confirm that the words used for the exercise were common across international, national and local documentation, and then presentation of the words during 24 focus groups using what was termed the "coffee" exercise to assess healthcare worker perception of commonly used words. In total, 2,000 health workers participated.

11.5 THE COFFEE EXERCISE

The premise of the exercise is concerned with word association, centred on the emotions and feelings evoked by certain words. Research has yielded powerful insights into how the brain mediates behaviour focused on mapping the semantic system (i.e. the meaning of language) within the brain (Huth et al. 2016). Most people across all communities feel some kind of instant emotion when thinking of the word *coffee*, whether it be energy or hatred. The exercise involved inviting participants to share, without discussing, the immediate feelings evoked from five words:

a) compliance
b) monitoring
c) alcohol-based handrub
d) system
e) moment

As participants called out their immediate responses, these were captured by the authors on flip chart paper until saturation or no more responses were offered. Quantitative analysis of the commonly evoked words was then undertaken.

During the exercises, approximately 240 words representing alcohol-based handrub were collected, 510 representing compliance, 402 representing monitoring, 480 representing moment and 200 representing system. *Compliance* in particular evoked negative feelings, with "cold words" being described on hearing this word, such as "policing," "difficult" and "punishment." A sample of the results for compliance is visualized in Figure 11.1.

The word *moment* evoked the most positive reactions ("warm words") such as *now, opportunity, time*. In summary, responses to the word *compliance*, with their overwhelmingly negative association, was not what the authors envisaged at the outset of the exercise. The findings have a number of potential implications for practice. IPC professionals should be visible and skilled in the art of communication as they seek to influence and engage colleagues in conversations on hand hygiene. In reality, is it the case that when health workers hear "We would like to talk about your latest compliance rates," what this stimulates them to immediately feel is a plethora of negative emotions that have potential to disengage rather than collaborate. A more recent conversation with the speechwriter specialist (Kilpatrick and Shovel 2021) revisited the topic, and the opportunity to explore new, more "warm" words that might engage health workers in hand hygiene improvement. This appears to remain an elusive goal.

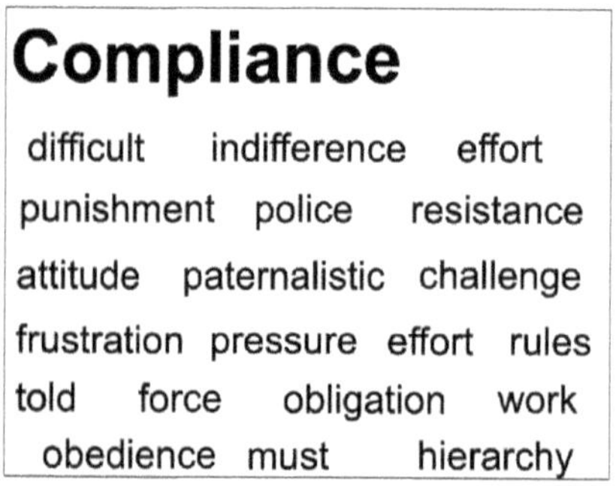

Compliance

difficult   indifference   effort

punishment   police   resistance

attitude   paternalistic   challenge

frustration pressure effort rules

told   force   obligation   work

obedience   must   hierarchy

FIGURE 11.1   Predominant feelings evoked by the word *compliance*

At the very least, co-production of hand hygiene initiatives with experts beyond the medical profession appears to be important going forward and has the potential to break down barriers between infection prevention and hand hygiene ideology and the reality of day-to-day clinical, and other, perceptions. This is particularly important if we are to make behaviour change, and as such improvement, a reality when as far back as 2009 WHO claimed that over the past decades there had been an inability to motivate health-care worker compliance with hand hygiene; we are now more than 14 years on. There will be prevailing linguistic nuances. However, (healthcare) processes are more efficient and are associated with more successful outcomes if all those involved base their approaches and communication on a common, positive language and therefore concepts. Addressing language alone may not lead to long-term behaviour change, but using an MMIS approach for hand hygiene and infection prevention improvement has been shown to be successful and should prevail (WHO 2017).

REFLECTION EXERCISE

Before reading on, think about the following;

1. The words used in your hand hygiene policies and guidelines, particularly in the context of measuring hand hygiene adherence. Is the word *compliance* used?
2. What does the word compliance evoke in you?
3. Do you talk about hand hygiene with your patients or clients? What words do you use?
4. If you have been involved in developing posters or promotional materials on any aspect of IPC, including hand hygiene—do you work with experts in any of the following areas: communications and marketing, behaviour change, human factors or any other of the social sciences?

11.6 CONCLUSION

It remains the case that IPC and hand hygiene practices continue to be suboptimal in many parts of health care in all parts of the world, which suggests that business as usual is not likely to work. Exploring novel opportunities that might change the status quo, including a focus on language, seems to be gaining traction. IPC competence in this area and the role of IPC practitioners as innovators in improvement approaches is more vital now than ever. Many of the words and terms used in association with hand hygiene improvement to date have been loaded with technical meaning, but they also have meaning as everyday words, and it is that dual meaning that can impact on what the audience hears when hand hygiene is communicated through guidelines, training, audit, advocacy and awareness raising.

Focusing on the words used in infection prevention in health care and their influence on human behaviour is still in its infancy. This is a journey of exploration and learning.

Building on the evidence that is available, IPC and academic communities have the opportunity to test their own audience's reactions to commonly used words, especially those featuring within policies and guidelines and even campaigns. The word *compliance* offers a logical starting point. Considering the relevance and potential benefits in developing a new taxonomy that breaks free of the current constraints imposed by a medicalized model, and one that draws on the science of behaviour change and neurolinguistics, now could be the time for a whole new way of influencing infection prevention and control in health care.

11.7 REFERENCES

Atkins L (2016) Using the behaviour change wheel in infection prevention and control practice. *Journal of Infection Prevention*, 17(2), 74–78. https://doi.org/10.1177/1757177415615952

Cole M (2014) Social construction of hand hygiene as a simple measure to prevent health care associated infection. PhD thesis, University of Nottingham. http://eprints.nottingham.ac.uk/14426/1/Final_PhD_revision.pdf accessed January 2022.

Crespo Fernandez E (2013) Words and weapons for mass persuasion: Dysphemism in Churchill's wartime speeches. *Text & Talk – An Interdisciplinary Journal of Language Discourse Communication Studies*, 33(3), 311–330.

Curtis V (2011) Why disgust matters. *Philosophical Transactions of the Royal Society of London. Series B, Biological Sciences*, 366(1583), 3478–3490. https://doi.org/10.1098/rstb.2011.0165

Edwards R, Charani, E, Sevdalis, N, et al (2012) Optimisation of infection prevention and control in acute health care by use of behaviour change: A systematic review. *The Lancet Infectious Disease*, 12(4), 319–329. https://doi.org/10.1016/S1473-3099(11)70283-3

Greene C, Wilson J (2021) *The Use of Behaviour Change Theory for Infection Prevention and Control Practices in Healthcare Settings: A Scoping Review*. University of West London. https://repository.uwl.ac.uk/id/eprint/3333/ accessed January 2022.

Huis A, van Achterberg T, de Bruin M, et al (2012) A systematic review of hand hygiene improvement strategies: A behavioural approach. *Implementation Science*, 7, 92. https://doi.org/10.1186/1748-5908-7-92

Huth AG, de Heer WA, Griffiths TL, Theunissen FE, Gallant JL (2016) Natural speech reveals the semantic maps that tile human cerebral cortex. *Nature*, 532, 453–458 http://gallantlab.org/huth2016/ accessed January 2022.

Huxley A (2007) *Brave New World*. Vintage Publishing.

Jumaa PA (2005) Hand hygiene: Simple and complex. *International Journal of Infectious Diseases: IJID: Official Publication of the International Society for Infectious Diseases*, 9(1), 3–14. https://doi.org/10.1016/j.ijid.2004.05.005

Kilpatrick C (2021) Something is not quite right in the pandemic messaging. *Nursing Times Opinion*. www.nursingtimes.net/opinion/something-is-not-quite-right-in-the-pandemic-messaging-28-01-2021/ accessed January 2022.

Kilpatrick C, Shovel M (2021, August 25) Mind your language. Infection control matters: Discussions on infection prevention. *Podcast*. Wednesday. https://infectioncontrolmatters.podbean.com/e/mind-your-language-with-claire-kilpatrick-and-martin-shovel/ accessed January 2022

Kilpatrick C, Storr J (2017) How we talk about hand hygiene matters—an exploration of hand hygiene etymology. *Antimicrobial Resistance and Infection Control*, 6(Suppl 3), I10.

Kretzer EK, Larson EL (1998) Behavioral interventions to improve infection control practices. *American Journal of Infection Control*, 26(3), 245–253. https://doi.org/10.1016/s0196-6553(98)80008-4

McClaws, ML, Sax H (2017) Behaviour and hand hygiene. In Pittet D, Boyce J, Allegranzi, B, editors. *Hand Hygiene: A Handbook for Medical Professionals*. John Wiley & Sons Ltd.

Mendelson M, Balasegaram M, Jinks T, et al (2017) Antibiotic resistance has a language problem. *Nature*, 545, 23–25. https://doi.org/10.1038/545023a

Michie S (2013) The science of behaviour change. In *Understanding Society, How Do We Change Behaviour*. Ipsos Mori Social Research Institute.

Michie S, van Stralen MM, West, R (2011) The behaviour change wheel: A new method for characterising and designing behaviour change interventions. *Implementation Science* 6, 42. https://doi.org/10.1186/1748-5908-6-42

Pearsall J (Ed) (2001) *The New Oxford English Dictionary*. Oxford University Press.

Simpson N (2021) Marketing 101- how to rebrand a fish. https://nicholashsimpson.medium.com/how-to-fall-in-love-with-a-fish-3b094432dd72 accessed January 2022.

Skinner H, Stephens P (2003) Speaking the same language: The relevance of neuro-linguistic programming to effective marketing communications. *Journal of Marketing Communications*, 9(3), 177–192.

Stolow JA, Moses LM, Lederer AM, Carter R (2020) How fear appeal approaches in COVID-19 health communication may be harming the global community. *Health Education & Behavior: The Official Publication of the Society for Public Health Education*, 47(4), 531–535.

Stone SP, Fuller C, Savage J, Cookson B, Hayward A, Cooper B, Duckworth G, Michie S, Murray M, Jeanes A, Roberts J, Teare L, Charlett A (2012) Evaluation of the national Cleanyourhands campaign to reduce Staphylococcus aureus bacteraemia and Clostridium difficile infection in hospitals in England and Wales by improved hand hygiene: Four year, prospective, ecological, interrupted time series study. *BMJ* (Clinical research ed.), 344, e3005. https://doi.org/10.1136/bmj.e3005

Storr J, Sax H (2017) Marketing hand hygiene. In Pittet D, Boyce J, Allegranzi B, editors. *Hand Hygiene: A Handbook for Medical Professionals*. John Wiley & Sons Ltd.

The Telegraph (2020, March 6) Boris Johnson sings happy birthday while washing his hands. https://youtu.be/EWfZGdLeDl4 accessed January 2022.

Wellcome Trust (2019) Reframing resistance: How to communicate about antimicrobial resistance effectively. https://wellcome.org/reports/reframing-antimicrobial-resistance-antibiotic-resistance accessed January 2022.

WHO (2017) Evidence of hand hygiene as the building block for infection prevention and control: An extract from the systematic literature reviews undertaken as the background for the WHO guidelines on core components of infection prevention and control programmes at the national and acute health care facility level. https://apps.who.int/iris/handle/10665/330079#:~:text=Evidence%20of%20hand%20hygiene%20as%20the%20building%20block,the%20national%20and%20acute%20health%20care%20facility%20level accessed January 2022.

WHO Guidelines on Hand Hygiene in Health Care (2009) www.who.int/infection-prevention/publications/hand-hygiene-2009/en/ accessed January 2022.

WHO SAVE LIVES—Clean Your Hands (2022) www.who.int/campaigns/world-hand-hygiene-day accessed January 2022.

Do Campaigns Make You Anxious? **12**

A Focus on Unintended Consequences

Julie Storr

Contents

> When I asked the doctor he looked at me as if I had two heads. I thought I was going to have a heart attack but forced myself to ask.
>
> (McGuckin et al. 2001)

12.1 INTRODUCTION

Storr and Kilpatrick (2015) in a review of campaigns and behaviour change highlighted the ongoing need to consider how messages are framed in relation to health care and public health campaigns in a world of potential message overload. Infection prevention

DOI: 10.1201/9781003379393-15

and control (IPC) has increasingly drawn on public health campaign insights, including the use of social marketing to achieve behaviour change and secure its intended impact of harm reduction and disease prevention. From a global perspective, Storr et al. (2016) presented a preliminary theory of change for IPC that aimed to ensure a strong convergence between efforts at preventing healthcare associated infection (HAI), including the associated costs, and other global threats from infectious diseases and the ultimate impact of achieving quality universal health coverage (UHC). Looking at this through an IPC lens, the desired long-term outcomes that would ultimately contribute to UHC included sustained health worker behaviour change, reduced incidence of HAI, reduction in antimicrobial resistance, prevention of avoidable harm and death and reduced risks of outbreaks of highly transmissible infections. One of the key IPC activities required at the global level in order to meet these outcomes was the use of campaigns and effective communication strategies, in particular a strong policy focus on social marketing and campaigning. This paper placed a spotlight on the IPC community's growing experience in this field.

The interrelationship between what IPC practitioners do and the quality of patient care is an important one. HAI is a well-known outcome measure in health-related quality of life research, and there is an increasing body of knowledge on the impact of HAI on patients' quality of life. Studies exploring the psychological impact of HAI have tended to focus on the impact of the infection itself and the interventions designed to interrupt transmission, such as patient segregation [isolation] and contact and other precautions. Results have been widely documented (Abad et al. 2010) with most studies highlighting a negative impact, including on higher scores for depression, anxiety and anger. Anxiety itself is an unwanted side effect of hospitalization because of the negative effects that it can have on patient's quality of life. However, little work has been undertaken addressing the impact on patient's health-related quality of life, of what might be termed nonclinical interventions, in this instance campaigns, designed to minimise the likelihood of HAI.

12.2 CAMPAIGNS AND THE PREVENTION OF INFECTION

Communications and campaigning in health care are rooted in the desire to influence human behaviour towards safer practices that will result in better outcomes. In an IPC context, outcomes should include not solely a reduction in the likelihood of HAI but improvements in the overall quality of life. Modern-day approaches in IPC build on decades of learning from wider public health/health campaigns, many of which were nationally driven in response to immediate and significant public health threats. The World Health Organization (WHO) presents a compelling argument for campaigning as a way of achieving global health improvement per se (Kilpatrick & Storr 2017). To illustrate this, WHO coordinates a global campaign on hand hygiene that takes place each 5 May. Drawing on the seminal work of Pittet and colleagues (Pittet et al. 2000), WHO's hand hygiene guidelines recommend the implementation of a multimodal strategy (WHO 2009). Use of a multimodal strategy now comprises the evidence-based core components of IPC programmes (WHO 2016). The strategy incorporates different constructs of behaviour change theory, including the health belief model (HBM) and the theory of planned behaviour (TPB) (Aboumatar et al. 2012) and is made up of five interrelated elements that address system change, training and education, monitoring and feedback, reminders in the workplace and institutional safety climate. The work of Pittet and later WHO to sensitise IPC practitioners to the power of such a strategy stimulated many (myself included) towards a shift from relying mainly on training, towards implementing many parallel endeavours, including campaigns, in the pursuit of sustained behaviour change. In addition to the global hand hygiene campaign, which was started in 2009, there are now a plethora of campaigns in IPC and related areas, including World Antimicrobial Awareness Week (Keitoku et al. 2021), World Sepsis Day (Schlapbach et al. 2020) and World Patient Safety Day (Binns & Low 2020). Each campaign has a strong advocacy component, aiming to both raise awareness and stimulate action. Evaluating the impact of global health campaigns is complex, and it is important to note that many hand hygiene campaigns remain under or unevaluated to this day (Kilpatrick & Storr 2017).

12.3 MESSAGE FRAMING

Kilpatrick and Storr (2017) summarise three key lessons from existing public health campaigns: (1) know and understand your audience, (2) have a clear and unambiguous message and (3) use the right media. How messages are framed (referred to in behavioural science as "message framing") is an important consideration if campaigns are to avoid what has been described as the boomerang effect. Counterproductive, or "boomerang," effects may be generated by media health campaigns (Atkin 2001) in which significant portions of the target audience are influenced in the opposite direction. In addition, a range of unintended outcomes are described within this phenomenon, including how the use of highly threatening messages may backfire without a strong efficacy component. Considering the HBM, Jenner and colleagues published an article that on the face of it critiqued hand hygiene posters. The paper included considerations of message framing and the use of fear as a tactic to influence behaviour, what the authors describe as "fear appeals" (Jenner et al. 2005). This fascinating study examined posters on hand hygiene promotion and how they were constructed within the context of message framing theory, whether they were considered persuasive, if the information was correct and consistent, to what extent fear appeals were used and the presentation style.

The authors describe a message as being a brief communication, either explicit or implicit. They focused on whether the messages presented in the posters were framed in terms of losses or gains, whether they applied the use of threats or fear appeals and the extent to which constructs such as personal responsibility as well as attitudes and perceived behavioural control were included. Less than half of those intended to motivate health workers conveyed messages that were "gain-framed," recognised in health promotion as how to frame messages positively. Mixed messages within posters were noted to be the inclusion of good and bad news. The authors noted that mixed messages may confuse rather than motivate. Forty-eight percent of the messages in the posters were neither "gain-framed" nor "loss-framed," with a note that this presents a lost opportunity and that posters were not being used as effectively as they could be. What jumps out of the paper is that "posters seldom drew on knowledge about effective ways to frame messages." It was concluded that more could be made of "repeated minimal fear appeals" but that messages should also be "gain-framed" and that "gain-framed messages" needed to be tested empirically. It is this testing that often fails to be addressed.

12.4 THE BOOMERANG EFFECTS, UNINTENDED CONSEQUENCES AND HEALTH CAMPAIGNS

In a fascinating article in the Guardian newspaper, Fleming (2022) states that in relation to health campaigns, "No matter how much groundwork policy wonks do, the risk of unintended consequences is always lurking." Fleming draws attention to a number of diverse campaigns to illustrate the point, two of which are focused on here. First, a paper on abstinence-based sex education highlighted that in the US, "increasing emphasis on abstinence education was positively correlated with teenage pregnancy and birth rates" (Stanger-Hall & Hall 2011). After accounting for socioeconomic status, educational attainment, ethnic composition of the teenage population, and availability of Medicaid waivers for family planning services in each of the states studied, these same trends were seen. The second case involves what has been described as "the sugary drinks levy" in the UK, in which soft drinks, high in sugar, are taxed—inflating prices for the consumer. One manufacturer of an iconic drink—Irn Bru halved the amount of sugar and replaced it with sweeteners to avoid paying the tax in an effort not to pass on costs to the consumer. The unintended consequences of this move not only included unhappy consumers but also a drink that now contained sweetening agents instead of sugar—agents that have been linked with a range of diseases. Fleming concludes by emphasising the importance of a multipronged approach that includes not just the policy lever itself but careful research of the target audience to aid in the development of effective communications, a deep understanding of culture and context, testing the intervention before widespread implementation and the need to routinely evaluate the impact of the campaign, including on unintended consequences and modify as required. Failure to address each of these elements can result in unintended consequences and contribute to the opposite of the desired effect.

12.5 SCARE TACTICS OR FEAR APPEALS?

Although not the main focus of this chapter, the COVID-19 pandemic highlighted some relevant insights into message framing, the use of fear and unintended consequences that will be briefly focused on, before turning back to campaigns employed during "peacetime."

In 2020, during the early stage of the pandemic, the UK government embarked on a campaign that could be described as using maximal or deliberate fear appeal, with one slogan stating: "CORONAVIRUS. Anyone can get it. Anyone can spread it. Stay home. Protect the NHS. Save lives" (HM Government 2020). The fear appeals, or what some describe as "scare tactics" (Stolow et al. 2020), worked in many respects. People did stay at home, and they protected the NHS, but in many instances, this meant not appropriately seeking treatment in a timely way due to fear. Payne cites a UK government minister in May 2021: "Our comms have been the best in Europe. We scared everyone shitless, but now we have to undo some of that." The strategy worked but had significant unintended consequences. For these reasons, Stolow et al. warned against the use of fear appeals in COVID-19 health communication, calling on decision-makers to employ evidence-based health communication, and in particular to consider local context and the needs of communities and then to provide practical, understandable information that supports the uptake of relevant behaviours. It is important to note that the authors do not underestimate the challenge for health professionals of developing and disseminating health communication messages in real time when there is uncertainty of evidence.

12.6 PATIENT EMPOWERMENT AS A CAMPAIGN STRATEGY

In a stark reminder that unintended consequences of IPC campaigns is a "thing," in one of the early studies into patient empowerment in the UK, a surgical patient's response to the question "Did you ask any healthcare workers to clean their hands" was "When I asked the doctor he looked at me as if I had two heads. I thought I was going to have a heart attack but forced myself to ask" (McGuckin et al. 2001). Inviting patients to participate in hand hygiene promotion however is now advocated by many organisations worldwide as part of their campaigns and strategies (Longtin et al. 2017). The WHO global hand hygiene campaign has periodically focused on patient empowerment as one of its annual themes. The use of patient empowerment as a campaign lever to drive health worker behaviour change is interesting when considering unintended consequences. Atkin (2001) states that most campaigns present messages that attempt to increase awareness, inform people what to do, specify who should do it and cue them about when and where it should be done but that all this comes with caveats.

The National Patient Safety Agency (NPSA) of England and Wales ran a national multimodal hand hygiene campaign during the 2000s: the cleanyourhands campaign. The campaign was pilot tested in nine hospitals for six months (NPSA 2004). One of the elements was patient empowerment and involvement (Randle et al. 2006). From the evaluation, 71% of patient respondents said that patients and the public should be involved in helping staff improve hand hygiene. The pilot also explored the unintended consequences of the approach. A broad theme reported by the patients interviewed was that a fear of consequences did put some people off asking health workers, "Have you cleaned your hands?" There were some clear parallels with that reported by McGuckin et al. from 2001 (see Box 12.1).

BOX 12.1   PATIENT-REPORTED FEARS AND
THE CLEANYOURHANDS CAMPAIGN

PATIENT FEEDBACK

- Would worry about how I would get treated by them.
- Would feel uncomfortable about doing it but would want to as it's my health I need to protect.
- Would not question because my care might be compromised.
- I wouldn't want to cause friction between myself and the members of staff looking after me.
- Take an awful lot of courage.
- You could offend them by asking.
- I think patients are frightened to ask staff if they have washed their hands because they might upset the staff or offend them.
- Patients fear that staff will treat them as a "trouble maker" or something if they were to ask staff to wash their hands.
- Many staff would resent it, and as a patient, the last thing you want to do is antagonise the staff.

To overcome some of these concerns, the NPSA undertook a further survey that included not only patients but the public and health workers, including IPC practitioners. Although not explicitly focused on unintended consequences, the findings were similar to previous studies, with a conclusion that further work was required to refute the myth among some health workers that patient involvement would undermine the doctor or health worker–patient relationship (Pittet et al. 2011). McGuckin et al. (2011) emphasised the importance of involving patients in the development stages of any programme to ameliorate concerns and challenges. The authors cite a study by Entwistle et al. (2005) in which the content of five leading patient safety directives in the United States was reviewed. They reported that the programmes had been developed without input from patients and lacked information about what health workers needed to do and what support should be given to patients.

McGuckin and Govednick (2013) suggest that the main emphasis of the academic debate has tended to address whether or not patients want to or should be informed and empowered, rather than the impact of encouraging empowerment on anxiety levels. And there has been little research that drills down into such an unintended consequence of a promotional campaign to empower patients, a point emphasised by Longtin and Pittet (2011), who stated that the impact of campaigns on patients' wellbeing and satisfaction deserves to be studied, calling for methodologically sound research on the topic.

REFLECTIVE EXERCISE

Before finishing the chapter, think back to the conclusions of Fleming and how these might be applied in your work. In particular, if you are involved in developing communications and messages as part of large or small-scale campaigns and initiatives, do you use a multipronged approach that includes any or all of the following:

- An edict from on high?
- Research on the target audience?
- Methods to consider the local culture and context (e.g. surveys, focus groups)?
- Pre-implementation testing?
- Post-implementation evaluation?
- Consideration of unintended consequences?
- Pause points to modify the approach based on post-implementation evaluation?

12.7 CONCLUSION

Atkin (2001) uses the word "safeness," meaning the avoidance of the risk of boomerang or irritation, as a critical consideration when considering how to convey health messages through campaigning. It appears that there is little research on "safeness" and the risks of boomerang or unintended consequences in relation to campaigning within an IPC context. This chapter briefly explored the role of campaigns in behaviour change and reflected on their unintended consequences, particularly whether campaigns to improve hand hygiene that involve patient empowerment make patients feel better or worse. This is an important consideration, and those interested in executing or researching the use of such campaigns should consider undertaking pre-implementation research of the target audiences and post-implementation testing to measure the impact of the campaign. In particular, further research to analyse the extent to which awareness-raising campaigns [particularly those that include an element of patient empowerment] to reduce HAI through improved hand hygiene compliance contribute to unintended anxiety in hospital patients would yield valuable insights. Given the increasing use of awareness-raising campaigns as a lynchpin of strategies to reduce HAI both inside health care and increasingly within the general population, this makes sense. Further research in this area would be valuable to ensure resources are utilized in the most effective and impactful manner and, at the very least, that they do not make people feel worse.

12.8 REFERENCES

Abad, C., Fearday, A., & Safdar, N. (2010). Adverse effects of isolation in hospitalised patients: A systematic review. *The Journal of Hospital Infection*, 76(2), 97–102.

Aboumatar, H., Ristaino, P., Davis, R.O., Thompson, C.B., Maragakis, L., Cosgrove, S., Rosenstein, B., & Perl, T.M. (2012). Infection prevention promotion program based on the PRECEDE model: Improving hand hygiene behaviors among healthcare personnel. *Infection Control & Hospital Epidemiology*, Feb;33(2):144–151.

Atkin, C.K. (2001). Theory and principles of media health campaigns. In Rice, R.E., & Atkin, C.K. (Eds.), *Public Communication Campaigns* (Third edition). Sage Publications Inc. Thousand Oaks, CA.

Binns, C., & Low, W.Y. (2020). World patient safety day. *Asia-Pacific Journal of Public Health*, 32(6–7), 300–301.

Entwistle, V.A., Mello, M.M., & Brennan, T.A. (2005). Advising patients about patient safety: Current initiatives risk shifting responsibility. *Joint Commission Journal on Quality and Patient Safety*, 31(9), 483–494.

Fleming, A. (2018). Unintended consequences: When government health campaigns backfire. *The Guardian*, Mon 16 Apr 2018. www.theguardian.com/lifeandstyle/2018/apr/16/unintended-consequences-when-government-health-campaigns-backfire Accessed Jan 6, 2022.

HM Government, England, public health campaign, 2020. www.gov.uk/government/news/new-tv-advert-urges-public-to-stay-at-home-to-protect-the-nhs-and-save-lives Accessed Jan 16, 2021.

Jenner, E.A., Jones, F., Fletcher, B.C., Miller, L., & Scott, G.M. (2005). Hand hygiene posters: Motivators or mixed messages? *The Journal of Hospital Infection*, 60(3), 218–225.

Keitoku, K., Nishimura, Y., Hagiya, H., Koyama, T., & Otsuka, F. (2021). Impact of the world antimicrobial awareness week on public interest between 2015 and 2020: A google trends analysis. *International Journal of Infectious Diseases: IJID: Official Publication of the International Society for Infectious Diseases*, 111, 12–20.

Kilpatrick, C., & Storr, J. (2017). National hand hygiene campaigns. In Pittet, D., Boyce, J.M., & Allegranzi, B. (Eds.), *Hand Hygiene: A Handbook for Medical Professionals*. John Wiley and Sons Inc. Oxford.

Longtin, Y., Sheridan, S.E., & McGuckin, M. (2017). Patient participation and empowerment. In Pittet, D., Boyce, J.M., & Allegranzi, B. (Eds.), *Hand Hygiene: A Handbook for Medical Professionals*. John Wiley and Sons Inc. Oxford.

Longtin, Y., & Pittet, D. (2011). Reply to "hand hygiene: Are we trying to make the patient the fail safe system?" *Journal of Hospital Infection*, 79(4), 380–381.

McGuckin, M., & Govednik, J. (2013). Patient empowerment and hand hygiene, 1997–2012. *The Journal of Hospital Infection*, 84(3), 191–199.

McGuckin, M., Storr, J., Longtin, Y., Allegranzi, B., & Pittet, D. (2011). Patient empowerment and multimodal hand hygiene promotion: A win-win strategy. *American Journal of Medical Quality: The Official Journal of the American College of Medical Quality*, 26(1), 10–17.

McGuckin, M., Waterman, R., Storr, I.J., Bowler, I.C., Ashby, M., Topley, K., & Porten, L. (2001). Evaluation of a patient-empowering hand hygiene programme in the UK. *The Journal of Hospital Infection*, 48(3), 222–227.

NPSA. (2004). *Achieving Our Aims—Evaluating the Results of the Pilot Cleanyourhands Campaign.* National Patient Safety Agency (Personal Copy). London.

Payne, S. (2021) Johnson seeks more sophisticated slogan to exit lockdown. *Financial Times*, May 1.

Pittet, D., Hugonnet, S., Harbarth, S., Mourouga, P., Sauvan, V., Touveneau, S., & Perneger, T.V. (2000). Effectiveness of a hospital-wide programme to improve compliance with hand hygiene. *Infection Control Programme. Lancet* (London, England), 356(9238), 1307–1312.

Pittet, D., Panesar, S.S., Wilson, K., Longtin, Y., Morris, T., Allan, V., Storr, J., Cleary, K., & Donaldson, L. (2011). Involving the patient to ask about hospital hand hygiene: A National patient safety agency feasibility study. *The Journal of Hospital Infection*, 77(4), 299–303.

Randle, J., Clarke, M., & Storr, J. (2006). Hand hygiene compliance in healthcare workers. *The Journal of Hospital Infection*, 64(3), 205–209.

Schlapbach, L.J., Kissoon, N., Alhawsawi, A., Aljuaid, M.H., Daniels, R., Gorordo-Delsol, L.A., Machado, F., Malik, I., Nsutebu, E.F., Finfer, S., & Reinhart, K. (2020). World sepsis day: A global agenda to target a leading cause of morbidity and mortality. *American Journal of Physiology. Lung Cellular and Molecular Physiology*, 319(3), L518–L522.

Stanger-Hall, K.F., & Hall, D.W. (2011). Abstinence-only education and teen pregnancy rates: Why we need comprehensive sex education in the U.S. *PloS One*, 6(10), e24658. https://doi.org/10.1371/journal.pone.0024658

Stolow, J.A., Moses, L.M., Lederer, A.M., & Carter, R. (2020). How fear appeal approaches in COVID-19 health communication may be harming the global community. *Health Education & Behavior: The Official Publication of the Society for Public Health Education*, 47(4), 531–535.

Storr, J., & Kilpatrick, C. (2015). *Journal Watch. Journal of Infection Prevention*, 16(3), 131–134. https://doi.org/10.1177/1757177415585594.

Storr, J., Kilpatrick, C., Allegranzi, B., & Syed, S.B. (2016). Redefining infection prevention and control in the new era of quality universal health coverage. *Journal of Research in Nursing*, 21(1), 39–52.

WHO. (2009). *WHO Guidelines on Hand Hygiene in Health Care*. World Health Organization. Geneva. www.who.int/publications/i/item/9789241597906 Accessed Jan 6, 2022.

WHO. (2016). *Guidelines on Core Components of Infection Prevention and Control Programmes at the National and Acute Health Care Facility Level*. World Health Organization. Geneva. www.who.int/publications/i/item/9789241549929 Accessed Jan 6, 2022.

Educating, Engaging, Campaigning—Social Media as an Adjunct to Infection Prevention and Control

13

Julie Storr, Annette Jeanes and Claire Kilpatrick

Contents

13.1 INTRODUCTION

Social media is ubiquitous. In 2021, over 4.26 billion people were using social media worldwide, a number projected to increase to almost 6 billion in 2027 (Dixon 2022). In a healthcare context, social media is firmly established as a mechanism of communication. In the preface to this book, we highlighted the UKRI description of social science as being concerned with the exploration of society related to the behaviours of individuals and the ways in which they influence the world around them, including the influence of general and social media on behaviours. Indeed, social media has been positioned by some as a matter of social science rather than technology (Solis 2012). On a global scale, the World Health Organization (WHO) and other health bodies working at a global level, such as the Centers for Disease Control and Prevention (CDC), use it as a mechanism to communicate health-related information to the public in a bid to influence behaviours. Many healthcare organisations and non-governmental organisations in almost every country have multiple social media platforms that are used to a similar end. It has a critical role in the rapid dissemination of information (Wong et al. 2020). Social media has grown as a method of communicating IPC information over the last decade, with McGuckin et al. (2019) finding that 14% of Americans surveyed stated they received their information on healthcare-associated infection (HAI) from social media. That such information is accurate and trustworthy is an important consideration, but this is not always the case (Moran 2020).

It therefore seems logical to include some reflections on the value that social media brings to the day-to-day work of IPC and consider some of the risks or unintended consequences. Indeed, is its potential to educate, engage and campaign being maximised? At the time of writing this book, there are scores of social media platforms. Based on the authors' experiences, this chapter will predominantly explore the answer to this question based on consideration of Twitter and YouTube; however Facebook, LinkedIn and Instagram are all used in an IPC context.

13.2 WHAT IS SOCIAL MEDIA?

Social media has many forms and is constantly changing. At a very basic level, platforms have been described as any media that facilitates social interaction. Wikipedia describes social media as interactive technologies that facilitate the creation and sharing of information, ideas, interests and other forms of expression through virtual communities and networks and lists a number of common features (Box 13.1) (Wikipedia 2022; Kietzmann et al. 2011; Obar and Wildman 2015; Boyd et al. 2007).

BOX 13.1   COMMON FEATURES OF SOCIAL MEDIA

1. Social media are interactive Web 2.0 Internet-based applications.
2. User-generated content—such as text posts or comments, digital photos or videos and data generated through all online interactions—is the lifeblood of social media.
3. Users create service-specific profiles for the website or app that are designed and maintained by the social media organisation.
4. Social media helps the development of online social networks by connecting a user's profile with those of other individuals or groups.

Readers excited to explore a graphic representation of the state of the social landscape are recommended to consult the Conversation Prism. The Conversation Prism (2022), a graphic chart of conversations between people on online networks, was created in 2008 by Brian Solis and JESS3. It is periodically updated in light of the continued evolution, spread and increasingly invasive nature of social media in people's lives.

13.3 SOCIAL MEDIA AND IPC

Literature on the use of social media in IPC is growing, and it is possible to find both academic and grey literature on its use in education and training activities, awareness campaigns, community engagement, risk communications during outbreaks, disease surveillance and pharmacovigilance (Madhumathi et al. 2021). These authors reviewed its use in the implementation of IPC practices and concluded that social media is the fastest and most efficient way of communicating with the general population as well as health professionals. They suggest it can help people take the right decisions and enable behaviour change—both critical for effective IPC implementation. Other studies have explored the use of social media as an adjunct to the dissemination of IPC research related to antimicrobial resistance (Cawcutt et al. 2019), as a method of engaging IPC conference attendees and the general public (Martischang et al. 2021), as a means of strengthening education (Lim et al. 2018) and as a mechanism for strengthening global and national campaigns, with a focus on hand hygiene (Pan et al. 2016; WHO 2022). It therefore seems apparent that it does have a potentially valuable role in protecting populations from the harms caused by HAIs and is worthy of exploration. Its role in disseminating evolving information during the COVID-19 pandemic is an interesting case in point (Patel et al. 2022).

13.4 EDUCATION-ENTERTAINMENT: YOUTUBE VIDEOS FOR HAND HYGIENE IMPROVEMENT

YouTube, a platform that enables video content to be shared freely, is ubiquitous. In the paper by Bora et al. (2018), according to internet traffic estimates, as of April 2017, YouTube was the second most commonly visited website worldwide. Information provided in the form of videos seems to be especially appealing to viewers of the internet and has been evaluated previously in relation to various health topics (Delli et al. 2016; Singh et al. 2012; Pandey et al. 2010; Nagpal et al. 2015). Particularly during epidemics, internet-based video platforms like YouTube experience a tremendous surge in viewer traffic, and therefore the potential for misinformation is real, as was demonstrated during the COVID-19 pandemic (D'Souza et al. 2020; Wong et al. 2020).

Bora et al. (2018) found that the proportion of videos containing misleading health information on YouTube to be sizeable, with 16.2% during the H1N1 influenza pandemic, 20.7% on West Nile virus infection, 30.4% on rheumatoid arthritis and 33% on hypertension. These authors found that when a query term is entered in YouTube with the default setting of "sorting by relevance," the YouTube search engine algorithm returns the results by measures of relevance after matching the metadata (such as title, short video description, keywords and tags/annotations that are needed to be furnished at the time of uploading) of the available videos with the query term searched for. They concluded that a particularly concerning aspect for public health information/communication was that even after being "sorted by relevance," a sizeable percentage of YouTube videos are misleading and inadequate. The study went on to find that a considerable proportion of the videos were misleading (approximately 25%). They were more popular (than informative videos) and could potentially spread misinformation. Videos from trustworthy sources like university/health organizations were scarce. During the COVID-19 pandemic, Li et al. (2020) found that over one quarter of the most viewed YouTube videos on COVID-19 contained misleading information, reaching millions of viewers worldwide. These authors called on public health agencies to better use YouTube to deliver timely and accurate information and to minimise the spread of misinformation.

Edutainment (education-entertainment) is a term that has gained in prominence in health care, describing the use of entertainment such as videos and games to support and fulfil an educational function. A randomised controlled evaluation study on the effectiveness of an edutainment video teaching standard precautions (the "Welcome on Board" video) by Wolfensberger et al. (2019) assessed learning effect (primary outcome) and satisfaction (secondary outcome) of watching a five-minute humorous edutainment video on standard precautions compared to reading a written standard operating procedure (SOP) or receiving no intervention. Edutainment was chosen

> as it is well known that emotions help learners to focus and facilitate uptake of information into long-term memory, we chose humour as the central emotional feature in this project. Positive emotions and the power of laughter can enhance the learning experience, and humour improves student performance by attracting and sustaining attention, reducing anxiety, enhancing participation, and increasing motivation.

The video was rated higher than the SOP regarding user satisfaction with the learning experience, and video participants more frequently indicated they would recommend this learning method to colleagues. They concluded that watching an edutainment video proved to be more effective to improve knowledge about standard precautions compared to reading an SOP or no intervention. Satisfaction with the learning method was superior in the video group, suggesting higher potential for future uptake.

Influenced by the growing use of education-entertainment as a communications strategy to inform, influence and shift societal and individual behaviours and the proliferation of entertainment-education YouTube videos focused on hand hygiene, two of the authors of this chapter collaborated with Lim et al. (2018) seeking to better understand the quality of these videos and explore the social media content and user engagement. A total of 400 videos were screened, with 70 videos retained for analysis. Of these, 55.7% (n = 39) were categorised as educationally useful. Overall, educationally useful videos scored higher than noneducationally useful videos across the categories of attractiveness, comprehension and persuasiveness. Miscommunication of the concept of "My 5 Moments for Hand Hygiene" was observed in several of the YouTube videos.

This study concluded that the availability of educationally useful videos in relation to hand hygiene is evident; however, it is clear that there are opportunities for contributors using this medium to strengthen their alignment with social media best practice principles to maximize the effectiveness, reach, and sustainability of their content. It is interesting to note that the work of Lim et al. preceded the growing use of podcasts as a social media for conveying IPC-related messages and information.

13.5 SOCIAL MEDIA IN THE REAL WORLD—IPC CAMPAIGNING

Social media is now widely employed in health-related campaigns as a form of social mobilisation (Chen and Wang 2021). However, in order to reach the intended audience, efforts must be targeted, and this is important if IPC campaigns are to influence behaviour and have an impact. The use of campaigns as one part of a multifaceted effort to improve hand hygiene is well documented, dating back to the early 2000s (Pittet et al. 2000; Gopal Rao et al. 2002; Storr 2005; Allegranzi et al. 2007; Matthai et al. 2011). However, many of these started in an era prior to ubiquitous social media use. As these campaigns have evolved, the influence of social media has grown, and reflecting on real world experiences in this arena reveals a number of key considerations and associated lessons. These might be useful for the reader who is keen to maximise the use of social media in their own local campaigning efforts—particularly in order to achieve success and avoid unintended consequences. A key message is the power of collaboration. Before embarking on a campaign, work with communications experts to understand the latest approaches and be prepared to start exploring campaign social media messages months in advance of the launch date. These considerations and associated lessons are summarised in Table 13.1:

TABLE 13.1   Considerations and lessons learned

CONSIDERATION	LESSONS LEARNED
Timing	• Give consideration to the exact times to issue messages on different platforms—if, for example, messages are being issued in support of a campaign day, issue them across different time spans within seven days of the campaign day. On the campaign day itself, depending on the topic, issuing approximately five messages is considered appropriate. Essentially don't peak too soon with your messages. Preparing others and issuing the actual messages to create a buzz across social media are two different things.
Target audience	• Consider your target audience. Messages should always be clear to all the public, not specific target groups. Also, ensure that key partners are ready to share your/similar messages; this will support your reach and amplify the message.

(Continued)

TABLE 13.1 (Continued)

CONSIDERATION	LESSONS LEARNED
Literacy and language	• The actual text which should be used within messages should always be understandable to the public, no matter what the intention of the campaign. Ultimately IPC should be aiming to achieve a healthier community overall, that is, the impact should always pertain to changes in public behaviour even if the campaign is thought to be targeted at IPC specialists. Facts and figures are always the most popular messages, but real-life stories and statements on the desired action going forward can also be impactful.
Colours	• Give consideration to colours used within campaign images—think branding and engagement. The use of more than three colours can be confusing.
Impact	• The intended target for each platform used should be clear from the outset so that evaluation of efforts can be assessed. Be clear on your ultimate goal. For example, on twitter it is impressions, on Facebook it is shares, on LinkedIn it is also shares, on Instagram it is likes. You might also want to consider sentiment analysis alongside quantitative analysis. And always be ready to consider competing stories/news—this can affect your reach but often cannot be planned for.
	• Develop a short- and long-term evaluation plan—a good place to start is the creation of a theory of change and SMART objectives, which will help keep the focus on inputs, activities and outputs. These can be evaluated more frequently than impact, which should be the ultimate consideration but will take a number of years, that is, agreed longitudinal data. Pre- and post-surveys are commonly used to address changes over time in target audience/public behaviours in relation to campaigns, and these can reflect your social media efforts. Using social media in support of campaigns is only one way of achieving impact.
Additional information	• Hyperlinks to further reading are commonly used in social media campaign messages—often campaigns have to keep their messages short and clear, but the intention is to drive people to a website to read more and, importantly, to use tools to take action for longer term impact.
Collateral	• Consider making available example messages and images for others to use—social media relies on a collective mass of people promoting the same messages for greatest reach and impact. Supporting people in this endeavour by providing pre-prepared messages is important. Similarly, calling for people to undertake a collective activity to support a message on social media can help your campaign, for example, a photograph or a commitment statement. However, be aware that the interest in such activities can change over time, and fatigue can occur.
Hashtags	• Appropriate use of hashtags—the use of hashtags changes. Be alert to the best use of these for your intended goal. For example, for broader reach, in recent years it has been considered that using only one hashtag is the best approach, but this can change.

Finally, before you start on your campaign social media journey, ask yourself, are you sure you have (or will have) the capacity to carry it through? Have you enough enthusiasm and energy to last for what could be a long haul? Is there enough information to say there is a need for a social media campaign, and are you ready to begin with the end in mind, that is, your intended long-term impact?

13.6 CONCLUSION

The studies, sites and examples reviewed seem to suggest that social media can be useful in IPC. YouTube videos on IPC appear to have great potential to be a useful source of healthcare information. However, there are some alarm bells to heed if the accuracy and trustworthiness of the content is not addressed. Just because something's easy and fun doesn't mean it is necessarily right and adds value. If we are to create and promote IPC-related videos on YouTube or any platform that might emerge in the future, IPC practitioners should be the trailblazers and leaders creating exciting, accurate, informative and entertaining content. Accurate health care information does not need to be dull either. WHO create excellent content on their YouTube channel that is evaluated well and helps save lives. Likewise, in the context of campaigns, social media is not going away anytime soon.

13.7 REFERENCES

Allegranzi B, Storr J, Dziekan G, Leotsakos A, Donaldson L, Pittet D. The first global patient safety challenge "clean care is safer care": From launch to current progress and achievements. *J Hosp Infect.* 2007 Jun;65 Suppl 2:115–123. doi:10.1016/S0195-6701(07)60027-9. PMID: 17540254.

Bora K, Das D, Barman B, Borah P. Are internet videos useful sources of information during global public health emergencies? A case study of YouTube videos during the 2015–16 Zika virus pandemic. *Pathog Glob Health.* 2018 Sep;112(6):320–328. doi:10.1080/20477724.2018.1507784. Epub 2018 Aug 29. PMID: 30156974; PMCID: PMC6381519.

Boyd D, Ellison NB. Social network sites: Definition, history, and scholarship. *J Comput-Mediat Commun.* 2007;13(1):210–230. doi:10.1111/j.1083-6101.2007.00393.x.

Cawcutt KA, Marcelin JR, Silver JK. Using social media to disseminate research in infection prevention, hospital epidemiology, and antimicrobial stewardship. *Infect Control Hosp Epidemiol.* 2019 Nov;40(11):1262–1268. doi:10.1017/ice.2019.231. Epub 2019 Aug 27. PMID: 31452490.

Chen J, Wang Y. Social media use for health purposes: Systematic review. *J Med Internet Res.* 2021;23(5):e17917. www.jmir.org/2021/5/e17917.

Conversation Prism 5.0 Brian Solis JESS3 graph. www.edigitalagency.com.au/social-media/conversation-prism-5-0/ accessed 21 Jun 2022.

D'Souza RS, D'Souza S, Strand N, Anderson A, Vogt MNP, Olatoye O. YouTube as a source of medical information on the novel coronavirus 2019 disease (COVID-19) pandemic. *Glob Public Health*. 2020 Jul;15(7):935–942. doi:10.1080/17441692.2020.1761426. Epub 2020 May 12. PMID: 32397870.

Delli K, Livas C, Vissink A, et al. Is YouTube useful as a source of information for Sjögren's syndrome? *Oral Dis*. 2016;22:196–201.

Dixon S. Number of global social network users 2018–2027. *Statista*, 15 Jul 2022. www.statista.com/statistics/278414/number-of-worldwide-social-network-users/ accessed 10 Jul 2022.

Gopal Rao G, Jeanes A, Osman M, Aylott C, Green J. Marketing hand hygiene in hospitals – A case study. *J Hosp Infect*. 2002 Jan;50(1):42–47.

Kietzmann JH, Kristopher H. Social media? Get serious! Understanding the functional building blocks of social media. *Bus Horiz* (Submitted manuscript). 2011;54(3):241–251. doi:10.1016/j.bushor.2011.01.005. S2CID 51682132.

Li HO, Bailey A, Huynh D, Chan J. YouTube as a source of information on COVID-19: A pandemic of misinformation? *BMJ Glob Health*. 2020 May;5(5):e002604. doi:10.1136/bmjgh-2020-002604. PMID: 32409327; PMCID: PMC7228483.

Lim K, Kilpatrick C, Storr J, Seale H. Exploring the use of entertainment-education YouTube videos focused on infection prevention and control. *Am J Infect Control*. 2018 Nov;46(11):1218–1223.

Madhumathi J, Sinha R, Veeraraghavan B, Walia K. Use of "social media"–an option for spreading awareness in infection prevention. *Curr Treat Options Infect Dis*. 2021;13(1):14–31. doi:10.1007/s40506-020-00244-3. Epub 2021 Jan 23. PMID: 33519303; PMCID: PMC7826144.

Martischang R, Tartari E, Kilpatrick C, Mackenzie G, Carter V, Castro-Sánchez E, Márquez-Villarreal H, Otter JA, Perencevich E, Silber D, Storr J, Tetro J, Voss A, Pittet D. Enhancing engagement beyond the conference walls: Analysis of Twitter use at #ICPIC2019 infection prevention and control conference. *Antimicrob Resist Infect Control*. 2021 Jan 25;10(1):20. doi:10.1186/s13756-021-00891-1. PMID: 33494810; PMCID: PMC7830043.

Mathai E, Allegranzi B, Kilpatrick C, Bagheri Nejad S, Graafmans W, Pittet D. Promoting hand hygiene in healthcare through national/subnational campaigns. *J Hosp Infect*. 2011 Apr;77(4):294–298. doi:10.1016/j.jhin.2010.10.012. Epub 2011 Feb 26. PMID: 21353722.

McGuckin M, Julie A, Storr J, Govednik J. Then and now (1989–2019): Patient empowerment and awareness of healthcare-associated infections, ICPIC 2019 poster presentation, 2019.

Moran P. Social media: A pandemic of misinformation. *Am J Med*. 2020 Nov;133(11):1247–1248. doi:10.1016/j.amjmed.2020.05.021. Epub 2020 Jun 27. PMID: 32603787; PMCID: PMC7320252.

Nagpal SJ, Karimianpour A, Mukhija D, et al. Dissemination of misleading information on social media during the 2014 Ebola epidemic: An area of concern. *Travel Med Infect Dis*. 2015;13:338–339.

Obar JA, Wildman S. Social media definition and the governance challenge: An introduction to the special issue. *Telecommun Policy*. 2015;39(9): 745–750. doi:10.2139/ssrn.2647377. SSRN 2647377.

Pan SC, Sheng WH, Tien KL, Chien KT, Chen YC, Chang SC. Promoting a hand hygiene program using social media: An observational study. *JMIR Public Health Surveill*. 2016 Feb 2;2(1):e5. doi:10.2196/publichealth.5101. PMID: 27227159; PMCID: PMC4869248.

Pandey A, Patni N, Singh M, et al. YouTube as a source of information on the H1N1 pandemic. *Am J Prev Med*. 2010;38:e1–e3.

Patel VR, Gereta S, Blanton CJ, Mackert M, Nortjé N, Moriates C. Shifting social media influences: Discussions about mechanical ventilation on Twitter during COVID-19. *J Crit Care*. 2022 Feb;67:191–192. doi:10.1016/j.jcrc.2021.09.017. Epub 2021 Oct 6. PMID: 34627649; PMCID: PMC8493479.

Pittet D, Hugonnet S, Harbarth S, Mourouga P, Sauvan V, Touveneau S, Perneger TV. Effectiveness of a hospital-wide programme to improve compliance with hand hygiene. *Infection Control Programme. Lancet*. 2000 Oct 14;356(9238):1307–1312. doi:10.1016/s0140-6736(00)02814-2. Erratum in: Lancet 2000 Dec 23–30;356(9248):2196. PMID: 11073019.

Singh AG, Singh S, Singh PP. YouTube for information on rheumatoid arthritis—a wakeup call? *J Rheumatol*. 2012;39:899–903.

Solis B. Social media is about social science not technology. *Social Media Today*, 15 Mar 2012. www.socialmediatoday.com/content/social-media-about-social-science-not-technology accessed 10 Jul 2022.

Storr J. The effectiveness of the national cleanyourhands campaign. *Nurs Times*. 2005 Feb 22–28;101(8):50–51.

WHO. World hand hygiene day 2022 unite for safety: Clean your hands, 2022. www.who.int/campaigns/world-hand-hygiene-day/2022 accessed 10 Jul 2022.

Wikipedia. Social media. https://en.wikipedia.org/wiki/Social_media accessed 10 Jul 2022.

Wolfensberger A, Anagnostopoulos A, Clack L, Meier MT, Kuster SP, Sax H. Effectiveness of an edutainment video teaching standard precautions—a randomized controlled evaluation study. *Antimicrob Resist Infect Control*. 2019 May 22;8:82. doi:10.1186/s13756-019-0531-5. eCollection 2019.

Wong A, Ho S, Olusanya O, Antonini MV, Lyness D. The use of social media and online communications in times of pandemic COVID-19. *J Intensive Care Soc*. 2021 Aug;22(3):255–260. doi:10.1177/1751143720966280. Epub 2020 Oct 22. PMID: 34422109; PMCID: PMC8373288.

Unshackling Infectiousness and Dismantling Stigma

Gay Men and HIV

14

John Gilmore-Kavanagh

Contents

14.1 SUMMARY OF KEY POINTS

- There are currently an estimated 38 million people living with HIV worldwide, but its impact on mental health and stigma remains a somewhat overlooked area in the literature—the emphasis of research has tended to be on prevention of transmission rather than the lived experience and all of its associated stigma.

DOI: 10.1201/9781003379393-17

- HIV transmission is more easily contained than other infectious diseases, but complexities around shame and stigma as well as the social exclusion of those who are most impacted are significant barriers to IPC. The history of HIV and AIDS is one of political controversy and turmoil.
- Public activism played a critical role in influencing policy and funding and putting a face to those impacted by the virus. This was in contrast to campaigns, some of which resulted in unintended consequences. Modern-day campaigns now empower rather than invoke fear.
- People living with HIV, on effective treatment, cannot pass on the virus (U = U). Therefore, focus on person-centredness of those living with HIV, effective treatment and barriers to treatment, such as shame and stigma, are in themselves public health and infection prevention and control measures.

14.2 OVERVIEW

HIV and AIDS have been topics of great interest in the domains of public health and infection prevention and control (IPC) for decades—and the scientific and social shifts in this area are remarkable. This chapter describes HIV and AIDS, primarily through the lens of the medical-sociohistorical significance of infectiousness and the associated impacts on HIV-related stigma and the psychological and emotional wellbeing of gay men as well as public health. The chapter further considers how in a new era of post-infectiousness in HIV, with the advent of pre-exposure prophylaxis (PrEP) and undetectable equals untransmissible science, this may work to dismantle societal and individual stigma and overall have a positive impact on the psychological and emotional wellbeing of gay men and the reduction of HIV transmission.

14.3 INTRODUCTION

Human immunodeficiency virus (HIV) is a virus that attacks the immune system. If left untreated, it can then lead to a person developing acquired immunodeficiency syndrome (AIDS), which is a collection of illnesses occurring because the immune system is so damaged it cannot fight off opportunistic infections. Discovered in the 1980s, the acquisition of HIV was a very serious health concern and in most cases led to death; however evolution of treatment means that now, HIV can be successfully treated, and while there currently is no recognised cure for HIV, those living with HIV and taking effective treatment can live a full and healthy life (Teeraananchai et al., 2017).

There are currently an estimated 38 million people living with HIV worldwide, and the majority are accessing appropriate antiretroviral treatment (UNAIDS, 2020); treatment means equivalence in life expectancy, but an issue which gets less focus in the literature is the impact HIV infection has on mental health and stigma (Lowther et al., 2014).

While there are people living with HIV in every demographic of society, the highest prevalence is found in women and girls living in Eastern and Southern Africa, as well as gay, bisexual and other men who have sex with men; stigma and mental health disparities are therefore complex and intersectional, in that these groups are likely to experience multiple forms of oppression simultaneously.

Gay men were the population in which the virus was first discovered and continue to be the most prevalent group within new diagnoses in much of the world. Gay men have also been at the vanguard of HIV and AIDS activism and lobbying since the 1980s—this brings a needed focus on the healthcare needs of gay men living with HIV, but so too it brings stigma and discrimination both outside of and within the gay community.

While HIV and AIDS have become very topical in areas of public health and IPC research, often the focus is primarily on prevention of transmission, a focus on HIV negative people and ensuring they remain negative. A shift in focus to the lives of people living with HIV, challenging stigma, and promoting mental wellbeing can have a significant impact not only on the individual's health but also on more engagement with healthcare services and adherence to medical treatment, which in turn ensures infection prevention techniques are adopted and new infections reduced.

14.4 AETIOLOGY

HIV belongs to a group of viruses called retroviruses; it has no DNA and contains all genetic material in RNA so cannot replicate itself. In order to make new copies of itself and grow, HIV RNA needs to embed itself into the host cell and use it to replicate new HIV cells. There are two strains of HIV identified, HIV-1 and HIV-2, with HIV-1 being the most prevalent.

HIV specifically targets the immune system by attacking its T helper or CD4 cells, white blood cells that are central in responding to infections in the body through the immune system, particularly the adaptive immune system. As these cells are killed off by the HIV, the body's ability to recognise and fight off opportunistic infections is diminished. Eventually this can lead to the development of serious illnesses in late-stage HIV, also known as AIDS. Treatment for HIV has developed over the decades, and now a combination of highly active antiretroviral therapies is standard treatment in disrupting various stages of the HIV life cycle. As well as keeping people living with HIV healthy by maintaining adequate CD4 counts, these drugs are also effective in keeping the virus at undetectable levels within the blood and therefore untransmissible—unshackling the infectiousness.

HIV is a blood-borne infection but also spreads through other bodily fluids, such as seminal fluid and to a lesser extent vaginal fluid, as well as breast milk; the majority of infections are through the presence of the virus in seminal fluid transmitted during sex through the mucous membranes of the vagina or rectum (Barreto de Souza et al., 2014) but can also be transmitted directly into the bloodstream—through the sharing of needles or through the infusion of infected blood products. The limited transmission routes mean that HIV transmission is more easily contained than other infectious diseases, but complexities around shame and stigma as well as the social exclusion of those who are most impacted are significant barriers to infection prevention and control.

14.5 SOCIOHISTORICAL CONTEXT

What we now recognise as HIV and AIDS were first recognised as a new disease in 1981 when growing numbers of young gay men were presenting with unusual opportunistic infections and malignancy, in the USA and later across Europe (CDC, 1981; Greene, 2007). Presented first as a "gay plague," it was coined as gay-related immune deficiency, and while its pathogenesis was not completely understood, it was established quite swiftly that transmission through sexual activity was a factor. The term AIDS was adopted in 1982, and it became apparent that the disease was not isolated to gay men. Throughout the 1980s a small group of scientists worked on isolating the casual link around AIDS, and in 1986 the newly identified retrovirus was named human immunodeficiency virus—HIV (Coffin et al., 1986). Retrospectively, HIV has been identified as far back as the 1920s, in Kinshasa, now Democratic Republic of the Congo, and demonstrates a cross-species transmission of simian immunodeficiency viruses from African primates (Sharp and Hahn, 2011).

Since their discovery, HIV and AIDS became established as areas of medical science littered with political controversy and turmoil. Politicians, policymakers and even medical leadership have often distanced themselves from what became one of the most prolific pandemics in history—HIV and AIDS are often met with negligence and denial. There are multiple instances throughout the last decades where funding has been withheld from HIV science endeavours, important policy documents blocked and an unwillingness to engage in evidence-based interventions, not only to prevent transmission, but also in the care of those living with HIV, including access to antiretroviral treatment and harm minimisation approaches to health promotion (Piot et al., 2007). While HIV and AIDS can affect anyone, where the most impact is seen is in those whom politicians and leaders are often seen to turn a blind eye: gay men, sex workers, drug users and those living in Southern and Eastern Africa. There is also a clear discomfort in many instances because of the very nature of HIV transmission—most transmission is through sex; shame and stigma prevail.

The inaction of governments and discrimination within society faced by people living with HIV was responded to with a groundswell in grassroots activism, especially within LGBT communities, led by people living with HIV (Wright, 2013). In 1987 the first chapter of ACT UP (AIDS Coalition to Unleash Power) was established in New York; this direct-action activist group was one of many, but perhaps the most visible and impactful. ACT UP chapters were formed across the world, and along with other groups, some very high-profile actions were carried out, to gain both political and public attention. The very public activism spearheaded by ACT UP and other community-led activist groups not only brought focus onto the issues around lack of funding and policy for HIV and AIDS but also "put a face" to those impacted by the virus. This was important at a time where public health campaigns around HIV and AIDS, operationalised and incited fear of the virus to combat transmission rates (Fairchild et al., 2018). Tactics of fear did little to inform the public around the actual risks of HIV, and these campaigns did little in terms of reducing transmission; while it may have been inadvertent, what these campaigns did do was further stigmatise people living with HIV and lead to HIV being weaponised in homophobia (Parker and Aggleton, 2003).

14.6 HIV TREATMENT AND INFECTION PREVENTION AND CONTROL TODAY

HIV treatment has developed significantly since the first drug AZT was developed in 1987; indeed the toxic effects of early treatment was in itself a barrier to providing safe and effective care. Currently there are more than 30 individual and more than 20 combination therapy antiretroviral medications available for treatment of HIV, many with minimal and very manageable side effects (Vitoria et al., 2019). The ultimate goal of these treatments is to disrupt the HIV reproductive cycle, reducing the virus to undetectable levels within the blood, so ensuring adequate CD4 levels for a functioning immune system. While a cure for HIV has not yet been developed, there have been reported cases of eradication of the virus following bone marrow transplant (Allers et al., 2010; Gupta et al., 2019) and remission from the virus—whereby HIV is not eradicated but controlled by the body's immune system without the need for antiretroviral therapy (Persaud et al., 2013; Heresi et al., 2020). There are also several ongoing studies aiming to develop a vaccination for HIV (Felber and Pavlakis, 2019).

Prevention strategies too have evolved. Condoms remain an important tool in HIV prevention, but the use of antiretroviral therapy as prophylaxis (PrEP) has emerged as a safe and effective HIV prevention strategy (Grand et al., 2010). PrEP has now become a mainstay of sexual health protection amongst gay men and, further to it, significantly reducing HIV transmission rates amongst communities where it is provided; PrEP has also been shown to significantly reduce HIV related anxiety amongst those using it (Keen et al., 2020). Furthermore, evidence has also emerged through the study of serodiscordant couples (where one partner is HIV positive and one partner is HIV negative) that people living with HIV who have undetectable viral levels cannot transmit the virus through sex (The Lancet, 2017). Public health campaigns are now shifting away from a fear-based approach, to empowering individuals through information, testing and access to condoms and PrEP. The issue of the use of fear and the unintended consequences of IPC-related campaigns is explored in detail in Chapter 12.

14.7 STIGMA

Stigma refers to the negative reactions experienced by individuals with a condition or characteristic which society deems as undesirable or discreditable (Goffman, 1963), and

HIV-related stigma has been identified as a key issue for people living with HIV and a priority for UNAIDS as they aim to eradicate the epidemic by 2030 (UNAIDS, 2015). The reasons that people living with HIV experience stigma and discrimination are complex and diverse and are often contextual and culturally specific (Mahajan et al., 2008). Indeed sources of stigma are multifaceted and intertwined. People living with HIV often internalise stigma while simultaneously experiencing that stigma from society, government, healthcare providers. A key driver of stigma surrounding those living with HIV is in the misinformation and ignorance around risks of transmission and fear of infectiousness through everyday interactions (Herek, 2002); this is further compounded by the negative attitudes around those most impacted by the virus, like gay men and sex workers. The complexity around stigma and HIV amongst gay men is multidimensional and cyclical; the experience of homophobia in itself is stigmatising. Stigma and discrimination then lead to oppression, which puts gay men at an increased risk of HIV infection; then the acquisition of HIV further compounds this stigma. Those who feel stigmatised have poorer access to health services, which in turn impacts their treatment adherence and indeed their physical and mental wellbeing, as well as their transmission-associated risks (Sayles et al., 2009). HIV-related stigma not only impacts those with a known HIV diagnosis but also creates hesitancy around testing, leading to late diagnosis and prolonged infectiousness (PHE, 2016).

The mental health impacts of HIV, while not solely caused by stigma, are very clearly linked. The experience of stigma is strongly associated with psychological distress (Stutterheim, 2011). People living with HIV demonstrate increased rates of anxiety and depression, and while the impact of HIV on physical health has been greatly reduced through treatment development, stigma prevails as a key precipitating factor (Lowther et al., 2014).

Despite the impact of stigma, not only on the individual living with HIV but also on public health and infection control measures, stigma reduction strategies are often not given the focus they require; they are relegated to the bottom of HIV prevention strategies almost as an add-on (Mahajan et al., 2008).

14.8 UNSHACKLING INFECTIOUSNESS

Anxieties around acquiring HIV amongst gay men are well documented; however, what gets less focus is the impact infectiousness has on the person living with HIV—fear of "passing on" the virus to a sexual partner, as well as a positive HIV status being a barrier to developing relationships (Stutterheim, 2011). Infectiousness and stigma therefore have a twofold impact; HIV negative people may avoid sexual contact with people living with HIV, leading to social exclusion, but so too people with HIV may have anxieties around passing on the virus to sexual partners who are HIV negative.

In this way, infectiousness plays a key role in narratives of stigma, and a focus on unshackling the concept of infectiousness from people living with HIV, a key strategy on ensuring stigma is reduced. The two most significant interventions here are the rollout of PrEP so that HIV negative people are confident in their protection from HIV infection, as well as "treatment as prevention" and U = U, promotion of testing so that HIV positive people are aware of their status, can receive prompt treatment and viral suppression to an undetectable level.

REFLECTIONS

Through focusing on a single infectious disease, this chapter raises multiple issues that perhaps are not as widely considered in the context of other infections. From your experience, do you think (a) the concept of infectiousness, (b) the narrative of stigma, (c) mental health impact on the patient are relevant in relation to the following healthcare-associated infections:

- Ventilator associated pneumonia
- Infections caused by organisms resistant to antimicrobials (e.g. MRSA)
- Pulmonary TB
- COVID-19

14.9 CONCLUSION

Undoubtedly, work will continue on "finding a cure" and vaccine development for HIV; scientific breakthrough in these areas would be monumental and have a massive impact on ending the HIV pandemic. But it is important to remember that we already have the tools to end the HIV pandemic today: widespread testing, condoms, PrEP and, most especially, effective treatment, as prevention are all strategies, which if adopted fully would lead to the end of HIV Transmission. While the end goal is an end to HIV transmission, this approach takes a shift of focus—from those who are HIV negative currently, onto those living with HIV. A shift onto unshackling the infectiousness of the HIV virus through viral suppression in people living with HIV. Indeed UNAIDS (2014) acknowledges the importance of treatment as a public health approach: the 90–90–90 targets set out to ensure 90% of people living with HIV worldwide would have a diagnosis through effective testing, 90% of people living with HIV would have access to effective treatment, and 90% of people living with HIV on effective treatment would be virally supressed. The 90–90–90 has the dual effect of ensuring those living with HIV live full and healthy lives, while concurrently ensuring that the virus is not transmitted to their sexual partners. While globally the 2020 targets have not yet been achieved, with ongoing focus on this approach, there is still a possibility to end transmission by 2030 (UNAIDS, 2020). This centring of people living with HIV foremost is a difficult task; remembering still today, those who are most impacted by the virus are often those most excluded; by unshackling infectiousness, we can dismantle at least some of the stigma these people face, and by dismantling this stigma, we can ensure more testing, more treatment and less transmission. Person-centredness on those living with HIV is also a public health and infection control strategy.

14.10 REFERENCES

Allers, K., et al. (2010) 'Evidence for the cure of HIV infection by CCR5Δ32/ Δ32 stem cell transplantation' *Blood* 117(10): 2791–2719.

Barreto-de-Souza, V., et al. (2014) 'HIV-1 vaginal transmission: Cell-free or cell-associated virus?' *American Journal of Reproductive Immunology* 71(6): 589–599.

Centers for Disease Control (CDC) (1981) 'Kaposi's sarcoma and Pneumocystis pneumonia among homosexual men-New York City and California' *Morbidity and Mortality Weekly Report* 30(25): 305–308.

Coffin, J., et al. (1986) 'What to call the AIDS virus?' *Nature* 321(6065): 1–7.

Fairchild, et al. (2018) 'The two faces of fear: A history of hard-hitting public health campaigns against tobacco and AIDS' *American Journal of Public Health* 108(9): 1180–1186.

Felber, B.K. and Pavlakis, G.N. (2019) 'HIV vaccine: Better to start together?' *Lancet HIV* 6(11): e724–e725.

Goffman, E. (1963). *Stigma: Notes on the Management of Spoiled Identity.* Englewood Cliffs, NJ: Prentice-Hall.

Grand, R.M., et al. (2010) 'Preexposure chemoprophylaxis for HIV prevention in men who have sex with men' *The New England Journal of Medicine* 363: 2587–2599.

Greene, W.C. (2007) 'A history of AIDS: Looking back to see ahead' *European Journal of Immunology* 37(S1): S94–S102.

Gupta, R.K., et al. (2019) 'HIV-1 remission following CCr5Δ32/Δ32 haematopoietic stem-cell transplantation' *Nature* 568(7751): 244–248.

Herek, G.M. (2002) 'HIV-related stigma and knowledge in the United States: Prevalence and trends, 1991–1999' *American Journal of Public Health* 92(2002): 371–377.

Heresi, G., et al. (2020) 'Sustained remission in a 4-year-old HIV-infected child treated in first year of life' Conference on Retroviruses and Opportunistic Infections, Mar 2020, abstract 347LB.

Keen, P., et al. (2020) 'Use of HIV pre-exposure prophylaxis (PrEP) associated with lower HIV anxiety among gay and bisexual men in Australia who are at high risk of HIV infection: Results from the Flux Study' *Journal of Acquired Immune Deficiency Syndromes* 83(2): 119–125.

The Lancet (2017) 'U=U taking off in 2017' *The Lancet HIV* 4(11): E475.

Lowther, K., et al. (2014) 'Experience of persistent psychological symptoms and perceived stigma among people with HIV on antiretroviral therapy (ART): A systematic review' *International Journal of Nursing Studies* 51(2014): 1171–1189.

Mahajan, A.P., et al. (2008) 'Stigma in the HIV/AIDS epidemic: A review of the literature and recommendations for the way forward' *AIDS* 22(Suppl 2): S67–S79.

Parker, R. and Aggleton, P. (2003) 'HIV and AIDS-related stigma and discrimination: A conceptual framework and implications for action' *Social Science and Medicine* 57(1): 13–24.

Persaud, D., et al. (2013) 'Functional HIV cure after very early ART of an infected infant' 20th Conference on Retroviruses and Opportunistic Infections, Atlanta, abstract 48LB, 2013.

PHE (2016) *HIV Diagnoses, Late Diagnoses and Numbers Accessing Treatment and Care.* London: PHE.

Piot, P., et al. (2007) 'Good politics, bad politics: The experience of AIDS' *American Journal of Public Health* 97(11): 1934–1936.

Sayles, J., et al. (2009) 'The association of stigma with self-reported access to medical care and antiretroviral therapy adherence in persons living with HIV/AIDS' *Journal of General Internal Medicine* 24(10): 1101–1108.

Sharp, P.M. and Hahn, B.H. (2011) 'Origins of HIV and the AIDS pandemic' *Cold Spring Harbor Perspectives in Medicine* 1(1): 1–22.

Stutterheim, S.E. (2011) 'Psychological and social correlates of HIV status disclosure: The significance of stigma visibility' *AIDS Education Prevention* 23(4): 382–392.

Teeraananchai, S., et al. (2017) 'Life expectancy of HIV-positive people after starting combination antiretroviral therapy: A meta-analysis' *HIV Medicine* 18(4): 256–266.

UNAIDS (2014) *Ambitious Treatment Targets: Writing the Final Chapter of the AIDS Epidemic.* Geneva: UNAIDS.

UNAIDS (2015) *On the Fast-Track to end AIDS by 2030: Focus on Location and Population.* Geneva: UNAIDS.

UNAIDS (2020) *UNAIDS Data 2020.* Geneva: UNAIDS.

Vitoria, M. et al. (2019) 'Current and future priorities for the development of optimal HIV drugs' *Current Opinion in HIV and AIDS* 14(2): 143–149.

Wright, J. (2013) 'Only your calamity: The beginnings of activism by and for people with AIDS' *American Journal of Public Health* 103(10): 1788–1798.

Physician Associates and Their Role in Reducing the Transmission of Infection—A Personal Perspective

15

Pam Trangmar

Contents

15.1 INTRODUCTION

This chapter is written from a very personal perspective and centres on the impact of a global health emergency on my day-to-day role. I am a physician associate and have worked in both a patient-facing role and an educational role, both within the National Health Service (NHS) and higher education, both before and during the COVID-19 pandemic, and although things have been difficult, there has also been joy in equal measure. Working in a busy hospital unit during the pandemic was a privilege and has shown the

DOI: 10.1201/9781003379393-18

best in the NHS, ranging from the cleaners to the consultants across an interprofessional spectrum. The amazing staff have really taken time to ensure that infection prevention and control (IPC) is on the top of the list for the patient, visitors and themselves, and I feel privileged to have been a part of this. The pandemic stimulated me to reflect on the fundamentals of IPC, and what follows is an account of this, culminating in a focus on the very essence of what IPC means to me—keeping environments, hands and equipment clean and safe.

15.2 IPC IN PEACETIME AND DURING TIMES OF CRISIS

At the start of the pandemic in 2020, my history consisted of working in hospital units/ wards for eight years, and pre-pandemic a key observation, both personal and backed up by the literature would be that hand hygiene compliance was not optimal (Lawson et al. 2021). This seemed to change during the pandemic with some improvement shown to occur (Wee et al. 2021). It is pleasing to see the positive changes that have happened over this difficult period. For example, from the literature, compliance with the required hand hygiene procedures appear to have improved during COVID-19, the pre-pandemic compliance being 54.4% compared to 92.8% during COVID-19 (Makhni et al. 2021). In the organisation in which I work, the need for reinforcing IPC policies took priority, and all the health workers that I worked with demonstrated exemplary hand hygiene techniques. The need to see patients, quickly and efficiently without putting anyone at risk is imperative, so adopting hand hygiene before and after interacting with them as well as the adoption of appropriate standard precautions for us all became essential practice (Adebayo et al. 2015; Hor et al. 2017). With the clinical setting, I am always conscious to ensure that I always adopt hand hygiene and other standard precaution measures where appropriate within sight of the patient to reassure them of my commitment to their safety.

COVID-19 certainly resulted in changes to the way we functioned in our hospitals. For example, I worked in a unit where the patients were tested for COVID-19 and, while awaiting the results, sat in chairs. Informed by the results, patients were then moved on to an in-patient ward, should they need to be admitted into the hospital overnight. Every bed space needs to be immaculately cleaned by the team of domestic staff assigned to deep-cleaning work to reduce as much as possible any risk of cross infection. I see patients that have come either from accident and emergency or via the ambulance service straight to the unit. This has its own difficulties as the situation with COVID-19 means that IPC measures must always be adhered to. Within my unit, the patients are all elderly so are also in a very vulnerable cohort of our society (Perrotta et al. 2020). Many patients present after an accident at home, which could have been caused by a variety of issues, including infections. When a patient presents, I will spend a lot of time learning what factors contributed to the patient attending my unit and finding out about their general health, living conditions and social environments. This means I will be working closely with the patient, and during this time I will also be examining them and taking any samples that may be required. Which also means that I will be exposed to potentially infectious organisms, and in turn, the patient is exposed to me, which serves to reinforce the fact that cross infection is a two-way process and is no respecter of boundaries within every conceivable environment. COVID-19 seems to have shone an intense spotlight on every aspect of IPC. Many of the interventions put in place to prevent COVID-19 spreading were in fact fundamental IPC practices which should have been happening anyway. COVID-19 intensified what should have been normal best practice, while clearly some additional measures were implemented due to the novel nature of the infection, the way it spread so rapidly and the many unknowns in the beginning. The ability to infect staff attending to COVID-19 patients was clearly felt early on, and the extensive personal protective equipment (PPE) policies were quickly developed. The ongoing need for face protection and gloves, even as the population has been vaccinated, has really enhanced IPC practices such as hand hygiene and glove use in all clinical and even personal environments. Unfortunately, as discussed by Makhni et al. (2021), there has been a gradual decline from a daily average compliance with hand hygiene of 92.8% (March 2020) in one hospital in Chicago to a pre-pandemic level of 51.5% in August of 2020 (Makhni et al. 2021). The paper does discuss this and acknowledges that there was a general fear around the start of the pandemic, and the admission into patient's rooms was greatly reduced during the highest infection levels, and the high levels of hand hygiene that is required has been difficult to sustain. As previously mentioned, on the unit that I have worked in, I have observed excellent hand hygiene with all patient-facing staff.

15.3 IPC—THE DAY-TO-DAY REALITIES

What does IPC mean to me on a day-to-day basis? First, I appreciate that it is vitally important that all members of the team are very thorough with regards to the fight against cross infection and that IPC procedures are carried out in accordance with guidance so that preventative practices are adhered to, and there is ongoing vigilance so that procedures are carried out safely. I understand that the environment in which care takes place can support people to do the right thing. For example, around the unit, there are gloves of various sizes, hand hygiene facilities and masks freely available. The access to these materials and infrastructures is vital for IPC to work.

However, in my experience I have found that the one area that is not addressed is the cleaning of what can be termed "personal fomites." A fomite is defined as an inanimate object that can be the vehicle for transmission of an infectious agent (CDC 2012)—items that are used, carried or worn within the work environment. For example, white coats are no longer worn as these were understood to be a carrier of infectious particles (Olise et al. 2018). In the UK, these were phased out, and it is now much more likely, during the pandemic, that you will see most patient-facing personnel in the areas I work in scrubs that can be laundered within the healthcare environment, so protecting the staff, the patients and the families of both from any infectious particles that may have settled on the clothing (Box 15.1).

BOX 15.1   THE CONTENTIOUS ROLE OF
UNIFORMS IN CROSS INFECTION

Health workers' uniforms continue to be the source of much study in the literature. A review from the UK in 2007 (Wilson et al.) tried to establish the current knowledge on the role of healthcare workers' uniforms as vehicles for the transfer of healthcare-associated infections. The review found that all components of the laundering process contribute to the removal or killing of micro-organisms on fabric. Furthermore, that there was at that time no robust evidence of a difference in efficacy of decontamination of uniforms/clothing between industrial and domestic laundry processes or that the home laundering of uniforms provided inadequate decontamination. Currently the significance of textiles, including uniforms, in the transmission of infection is not entirely clear (Owen & Laird 2020). Pathogens may survive the laundering process, and a significant area of concern is the potential for inadequate domestic laundering (Honisch et al. 2014), though industrial laundering of uniforms may also be inadequate (Chiereghin et al. 2020). The COVID-19 pandemic led to an increase in the provision of centralised laundering of uniforms in many organisations, which was in part related to the recognition of the potential risk of home laundering.

Other fomites that I have noted being used are pens, stethoscopes, mobile phones, desk telephones and computers. Working on a busy unit means that extra care is needed to ensure that these items are cleaned every time that they are used. Unfortunately, this is not always the case as the demands on the staff due to equipment shortages and workloads means that the need to work as quickly and efficiently whilst remaining vigilant to one's own practice and the practice of colleagues in relation to the risks of cross infection. In my personal experience, this is an aspect of practice that is not well recognised or emphasised within the context of caring for the carers, which on occasion is sorely missing. This raises important issues in relation to awareness of risks, training and communication—all important in influencing the behaviour and practice of health workers. I will expand on these later.

Within the practice setting, it is perceived as being acceptable to see stethoscopes hanging around the necks of the clinicians, pens in the pocket with the ever-available mobile telephone (Siddqui et al. 2018). When it comes to the fomites that we all carry, I also feel it is important to carry a saturation monitor with me, the importance of which increased due to the COVID-19 pandemic. It always needs to be remembered that infectious particles can be on any item that practitioners or patients have touched. With the following in mind, where IPC is concerned, it is vital that such cleaning becomes second nature to all. Although I do this myself, I recognise and am motivated with regards to IPC the need to keep all these items clean (Siddiqui et al. 2018). All my colleagues and I have been trained in IPC and am aware of the guidelines and try to keep up to date.

My perception is that patients never seem to be aware of this, and I have never been asked for example if these items are clean (Juraja 2013). What I find interesting is that in contrast, I have been asked whether my hands are clean, which is something that should be encouraged among patients, but what about other potential sources of cross infection? It is clear that a great deal of emphasis has been placed on hand hygiene improvement—which I do not disagree with—but now is perhaps the time to rebalance this with a parallel focus on other areas, including fomites and the importance of cleaning and decontamination of these (Peters et al. 2018).

Moving from awareness to action takes a multipronged approach. Policies and guidance are one important part of driving safe practice. With regard to stethoscopes, within my unit, effective and medically appropriate wipes are used to keep this important instrument safe. Such wipes regarding the cleansing of equipment carried by a practitioner must be placed in highly visible locations and where the dispensers are easily accessible. This is a matter of human factors and is covered in more detail in Chapter 10. Detergent/disinfectant wipes work well on both personal fomites but also the plastic chairs, side tables and blood pressure cuffs commonly found in hospitals. As a part of my role, I am vigilant in ensuring that all the clinicians I work with clean their own stethoscopes, and because of this it is becoming a more normalised routine. The power of motivated health workers to influence colleagues cannot be underestimated—the term *role models* is often used to describe such people. I try to role model best practices to influence colleagues to practice effective IPC.

Other common pieces of equipment that are highly touched and used by multiple workers include computers. Once I have met with the patient, I need to type up my findings, which means using a computer. Our computers are within the unit and have a plastic-coated keyboard, which enables cleaning to be undertaken after every use—again, this is a design feature to support cleaning. As part of my role modelling and leading role championing IPC, I clean computers when I, along with another colleague, get to the unit in the morning. A recent systematic review undertaken by Ide et al. (2019) reports that there is not a clear link between device contamination and healthcare/patient infections even though contamination of keyboards ranged from 23% to 100% with such pathogens as methicillin-resistant *Staphylococcus aureus*, *Clostridium difficile*, vancomycin-resistant *Enterococci* and *Escherichia coli*. (Ide et al. 2019). Importantly, gloves are not encouraged to be worn at the keyboard; rather, workers are advised to undertake hand hygiene before touching the keyboard to ensure any microbes from the last patient or surface touched are removed/destroyed. I can confidently say that within my unit, this is undertaken by my colleagues as a routine action.

Some fomites do not tend to receive as much attention. How important is it, for example, that pens are not so routinely wiped down and telephones hardly at all? There is some evidence that these can be vectors for cross infection (Curtis et al. 2018). The fact that working on the unit, which is likely to be heavily contaminated with potentially infectious microbes, is a strong motivator to consider telephones and pens and the need to clean them frequently. The day-to-day reality for me (and therefore for many colleagues) is as follows: I use my phone to keep in contact with my colleagues through online meeting platforms such as Microsoft Teams or Zoom and also to look up medication on the latest version of the British National Formulary App (BNF/NICE). This means that the phone is in use for a large percentage of the day—constantly being touched by my hands and why I believe even though I am sure I perform timely hand hygiene, there is still the chance for my phone to be contaminated, and so it is important to regularly clean it. Our perceptions are important to us and influence our behaviours.

My observations of others reveal interesting behaviours. There are times that I note colleagues walk away from having touched a patient, sometimes with gloved hands, and they are using their mobile phones. The phone then slips back into the pocket, contaminated and unclean. An IPC anomaly. This less-than-ideal practice can be exacerbated by pressures of work which contribute to lapses of vigilance. However, this is where, as indicated previously, each of us needs to be vigilant of our colleagues and to step in to support them as role models and mentors when such lapses of infection control practice occur. Supporting each other, modelling best practice and caring for the carers is vital.

Finally, as this chapter draws to a close, it is important to remember that IPC is all about human behaviours and that patients also have a role to play. I see patients with pens up against their faces and mouths, and then they put them down on the table whilst completing a form or the crossword. Role modelling and feedback is not something that should be confined solely to our colleagues but to patients and relatives also. There is also the need to support and educate patients about the risks of infection and the potential for cross infection. Most patients are interested in IPC, and they understand that they are also helping themselves as well as us. Cleaning pens in a healthcare environment is potentially important (Patil et al. 2010). In consideration of this, it is worth taking the time to clean fomites thoroughly before leaving your place of work. COVID-19 heightened our awareness of the importance of fomites and cleaning, but a clean, safe environment in health care is important to protect patients and workers from a whole range of potentially harmful microbes.

As I reflect on the reality of IPC in the area I work, if I were asked to list the top ingredients that contribute to good practices, I would list the following: (1) robust guidance/ policies and awareness of their existence; (2) leadership and role modelling across the trust that values IPC, including my development as a role model and the pride I feel in helping to keep others safe; (3) a training programme that helps support implementation of guidance.

15.4 CONCLUSION

In conclusion, this chapter has been my journey through IPC in my area of work, and I hope that some of the points raised will be standards that can be taken forward and adopted in other clinical environments. The need for fomites to be included in regular cleaning routines by the individual is important but is easily overlooked. Encouraging each clinician, nurse and healthcare assistant to take control of their own equipment, whether it is their stethoscope, phone or pen, should be an aim that we can all achieve. Patients come to us with hope that they will get the treatment that they require, and this should be without the fear of contracting a nosocomial infection from easily cleaned personal items.

15.5 REFERENCES

Adebayo, O., Labiran, A., Imarhiagbe, L. Standard precautions in clinical practices: A review. *IJHSR*. 2015;5:521–528.

BNF British National Formulary—NICE. https://bnf.nice.org.uk.

Center for Disease Control and Prevention (CDC). *Principles of epidemiology in public health practice, 3rd ed: An introduction to applied epidemiology and biostatistics.* Washington, DC: Public Health Foundation, 2012.

Chiereghin, A., Felici, S., Gibertoni, D., Foschi, C., Turello, G., Piccirilli, G., Gabrielli, L., Clerici, P., Landini, M., Lazzarotto, T. Microbial contamination of medical staff clothing during patient care activities: Performance of decontamination of domestic versus industrial laundering procedures. *Curr. Microbiol.* 2020;77(7):1159–1166.

Curtis, A., Moore, Z., Patton, D., O'Connor, T., Nugent, L. Does using a cellular mobile phone increase the risk of nosocomial infections in the neonatal intensive care unit: A systematic review. *J Neonatal Nurs.* 2018 Jun 1;24. doi: 10.1016/j.jnn.2018.05.008.

Honisch, M., Stamminger, R., Bockmühl, D.P. Impact of wash cycle time, temperature and detergent formulation on the hygiene effectiveness of domestic laundering. *J. Appl. Microbiol.* 2014;117:1787–1797.

Hor, S., Hooker, C., Iedema, R., et al. Beyond hand hygiene: A qualitative study of the everyday work of preventing cross-contamination on hospital wards *BMJ Quality & Safety.* 2017;26:552–558.

Ide, N., Frogner, B.K., LeRouge, C.M., et al. What's on your keyboard? A systematic review of the contamination of peripheral computer devices in healthcare settings. *BMJ Open.* 2019;9:e026 437. doi: 10.1136/bmjopen-2018-026437.

Juraja, M. *The Patient's Perception of Infection Prevention and Control in Healthcare.* Australia: Hospital and Healthcare, Westwick-Farrow Media. 2013. www.hospitalhealth.com.au/con tent/clinical-services/news/the-patients-perception-of-infection-prevention-and-control-in-healthcare-1404353893.

Lawson, A., Vaganay-Miller, M., Cameron, R. An investigation of the general population's self-reported hand hygiene behaviour and compliance in the cross-European setting. international. *JERPH.* 2021;18:2402. https://doi.org/10.3390/ijerph18052402.

Makhni, S., Umscheid, C.A., Soo, J., et al. Hand hygiene compliance rate during the COVID-19 pandemic. *JAMA Intern Med.* 2021;181(7):1006–1008. doi: 10.1001/jamainternmed.2021.1429.

Olise, C.C., Simon-Oke, I.A., et al. Fomites: Possible vehicle of nosocomial infections. *J Pub Health Catalog.* 2018;1(1):16–16. doi: 10.35841/public-health-nutrition.1.1.11–16

Owen, L., Laird, K. The role of textiles as fomites in the healthcare environment: A review of the infection control risk. *Peer J. Life Environ.* 2020;25(8):e9790.

Patil, P., Hulke, S., Avinash, T., Gaikwad, M. Pen of health care worker as vector of infection. *OJHAS.* 2010 Jul 1;9(3).

Perrotta, F., Corbi, G., Mazzeo, G. et al. COVID-19 and the elderly: Insights into pathogenesis and clinical decision-making. *Aging Clin Exp Res.* 2020;32:1599–1608. https://doi.org/10.1007/s40520-020-01631-y.

Peters, A., Otter, J., Moldovan, A., et al. Keeping hospitals clean and safe without breaking the bank: Summary of the healthcare cleaning forum 2018. *Antimicrob Resist Infect Control.* 2018;7(132):2020.

Siddiqui, S., Jamal, H., Kotgire, S., Afreen, U. Bacterial contamination of mobile phones of healthcare workers at a tertiary care hospital. *Indian J Microbiol Res.* 2018;5(4):460–465.

Wee, Liang En Ian, et al. Unintended consequences of infection prevention and control measures during COVID-19 pandemic. *Am J Infect Control.* 2021;49(4):469–477. ISSN 0196–6553, https://doi.org/10.1016/j.ajic.2020.10.019.

Wilson, J.A., Loveday, H.P., Hoffman, P.N., Pratt, R.J. Uniform: An evidence review of the microbiological significance of uniforms and uniform policy in the prevention and control of healthcare-associated infections. *Report to the Department of Health (England). J Hosp Infect.* 2007 Aug;66(4):301–307. doi: 10.1016/j.jhin.2007.03.026. Epub 2007 Jun 28. PMID: 17602793.

Infection Prevention and Control in Healthcare-Built Environments

16

Annette Jeanes

Contents

16.1 BACKGROUND

It is accepted that the environment has a general role in the transmission and acquisition of infection (Suleyman et al. 2018). The design of facilities, cleanliness, disinfection, ventilation, maintenance, management of waste and isolation provision in the healthcare environment have all been recognised as important in reducing the risk of infection (Dancer 2014; Olmsted et al. 2016; O'Connell & Humphreys 2000). Opportunities to improve the environment to control and reduce infection have been acknowledged, and this is a developing

DOI: 10.1201/9781003379393-19

area. Undertaking environmental research in functioning healthcare facilities is, however, challenging, and the available evidence base is limited and may be undermined by a lack of controls and the presence of variables. Fortunately, evidence from other disciplines can be utilised in health care (Ulrich et al. 2008).

More recently the specific effects of the built healthcare environment on aspects relevant to IPC such as people's behaviour, health outcome and infection prevention and control practices have been recognised (Tanja-Dijkstra & Pieterse 2011; Huisman et al. 2012).

16.2 INFECTION PREVENTION AND CONTROL ROLE

The time and effort required by infection control practitioners (ICPs) to ensure the physical environment of health care is optimal is often underestimated. IPC support and input is required at many levels and spheres, including planning, building, maintenance and identifying barriers to IPC compliance and opportunities for improvement. Infection control advisors must also ensure that organisations are aware of mandatory infection control requirements and guidance, including safe water supply, air exchanges, space requirements and risk assessment for demolition and preparation of the areas for redevelopment (Stockley et al. 2006).

When the environment of health care potentially increases the risk of infection and transmission, the role of the ICP is to identify, report and where possible mitigate the potential risk and seek assistance. When the ICP recognises the advice required is beyond their expertise, it is accepted that they may require the support of "superspecialists," that is, those with in-depth knowledge such as hospital ventilation. ICPs are neither omnipotent nor omnipresent and may miss environmental issues of concern, which is why the support of colleagues is important.

An essential part of the ICP role is to be a visible presence and to actively experience the healthcare environment. This includes audit, monitoring and risk assessments, though a simple audit may not understand the potential consequences of what happens in practice. It is also useful to simply be there to observe or seek feedback. This is a valuable use of time as an expert may identify more than a casual observer (Persky & Robinson 2017).

Example 1: The ICP observes the sharps disposal bin has been placed on the wall two meters behind the phlebotomist/venepuncturists workstation. To dispose of a sharp/used syringe and needle immediately the phlebotomist/venepuncturist must turn and walk across the space to place it in the bin. Instead, they recap the sharp instrument and/ or just place them in a receptacle for later disposal, which increases the risk of injury.

Example 2: An ICP and a clinician entered a clinical area, and the ICP attempted to clean their hands at the sink. The soap dispenser didn't seem to work. The clinician steps forward and said, "It doesn't work like that. You must reach inside and milk the tube inside as the button has fallen off." The ICP subsequently found that approximately 20% of the soap dispensers were broken in the facility.

Other useful approaches may include observations made while following the patient or visitors' journey through a hospital, including to the visitors' toilets, reception and waiting areas. Visitors may be acutely aware of the state of the environment, including the smell, the noise and out-of-date information posters but may not comment. Seeing and reporting chipped paint, dirty vents, dusty rails and broken equipment stored in a corridor may not be popular but will highlight the continuous need to maintain an optimal environment for infection control purposes.

16.3 FRESH EYES AND AGENTS FOR CHANGE

The use of "fresh eyes" in IPC is important as people who regularly inhabit a work environment may become blind to the conditions and no longer notice shortcomings. Staff focused on getting the job done may miss something significant, as demonstrated by the selective attention experiments by Simons and Chabris (1999).

Whilst it may be assumed that new staff coming into the environment will notice and report problems, this may not happen and may also be influenced by cultural and contextual factors. In a study of nurses entering a new workplace in Korea, Kim et al. (2016) found that there were unspoken rules of not criticising the environment and how things were done as many established staff did not welcome criticism. This was particularly challenging for experienced members of staff going into a new workplace environment as it was assumed that they knew the rules and would not criticise to gain acceptance.

Kim describes "going silent" as a strategy to survive the initial phase of working in a new environment as it is less stressful and allows time to learn what is acceptable. This process of assimilation may then lead to an acceptance of the environment and behaviours as the norm, and initial criticisms may be lost. There may be a similar response following the transition shock that medical students and nurses experience when moving from university, where they are taught what should happen, to hospitals, where they encounter what actually happens (Wakefield 2018). There is a general aversion to rocking the boat and a preference for wanting to fit in particularly when the response is that "it's always like this."

It is particularly problematic if someone is brave enough to speak up and voice an opinion on the environment and nothing changes as such efforts may be perceived to be futile, and instead the person is labelled as negative or deviant.

Despite an initial discomfort with an environment, people often may come to terms with it by a process of cognitive dissonance (Brehm & Cohen 1962), whereby they either become ambivalent or find other positive aspects which they like. This acceptance of the way things are and a lack of critical scrutiny may allow problems to get worse and are then more difficult to resolve.

Cleaning and maintenance staff have a unique perspective of the healthcare environment and are a source of information (Chen & Skillen 2006). Their recognition of what does and doesn't work, what's wearing out or frequently broken, how problems could be resolved and other solutions are based on practical experience (Jeanes et al. 2012). This may be particularly relevant for discovering workarounds (Jeanes et al. 2018).

Example: In one area there were frequent complaints of overflowing waste bins, which was attributed to the new waste bags being stored in a cupboard only accessible to cleaning staff. This was not a problem in another area as clinical staff kept a secret supply of such bags and other potentially useful stores in a cupboard only accessible by them.

16.4 THE EXPERIENCE OF THE PATIENT

The subjective experience of patients using healthcare facilities is an important factor in ensuring positive outcomes of care. The operational efficiency, quality of caring and physical environment, all contribute to the experience of individuals dealing with illness.

Whilst the design of healthcare facilities may influence infection transmission, length of stay and stress (Edvardsson et al. 2008), the physical environment may also exacerbate the stress and anxiety which the patient or visitor is already experiencing in their healthcare journey, particularly in an unfamiliar environment. Initial impressions of health care usually focus more on interactions with carers and staff rather than the environment (Brownall et al. 2013), but perceptions of the environment can affect expectations of standards of care (Douglas & Douglas 2005).

Time alone or waiting allows patients and their carers time to consider the environment of care. Some groups, such as healthcare professionals, may be able to rationalise some of the risks of transmission from the environment and behaviours, which they encounter (Dancer 2012). Whilst others may be concerned that corridors are untidy, that there is a small quantity of dried blood splatter on the floor or that their possessions are not secure when they go for tests. A quiet, orderly and clean environment may give the impression of a safe and secure environment, whilst a noisy, untidy and dirty environment may give the initial impression of a chaotic and unsafe environment.

Although these impressions may be misleading, they can influence the response of the patient of their subsequent care and become self-fulfilling prophesies (Jussim 1986). This bias in opinion may affect the subsequent trust of patients and their willingness to adhere to recommended treatments.

Example: I knew I would get an infection as the floor was dirty, the toilets were smelly and the furniture was scruffy.

What happens to patients or clients using a healthcare facility may be beyond their control, for example: How long will I have to wait? What will happen? Will it be painful? What will test results show? Some of the anxiety and stress can be eased where possible by enabling patients some level of control of the environment. This may include the level of noise, light, temperature or ventilation, which can help to normalise their environment. This assumes that the person has the capacity or courage to express their preferences and may not be an option, particularly on a short visit, but which may cause continuing stress when endured for long periods. Examples include lack of access to hand hygiene facilities prior to eating, draughts from open windows, inability to use their own pillow or bedding.

Unfortunately, many patients have a fear of alienating themselves and may avoid expressing their views to HCWs (Burnett et al. 2010), and consequently their preferences may not be recognised or may not be possible. An example is the provision of single rooms, which are often preferred by patients (Maben et al. 2016), particularly to provide privacy but may be in short supply, whilst patients may have little choice when they are required to isolate. In this example, a compromise of optimal provision of single rooms and the provision and design of facilities to enable communication with the outside world and avoid disorientation is required.

The results of a study by Huisman et al. 2012 of the impact of physical environmental factors on users suggested that the healing process was affected by the physical environment. Aspirations to achieve a healing environment, as suggested by the work of Ulrich (1992), have influenced healthcare planning. However, there is limited evidence that both patient and staff requirements or concerns are fully considered when determining benefits. A problem of enabling more control of the environment for patients to make choices and feel more relaxed is a lack of uniformity, loss of control for staff and sometimes the introduction of unnecessary risks. Variations in, for example, when the lights are turned on may conflict with staff expectations and affect the routines such as cleaning times, ward rounds, mealtimes. There are benefits of standardisation of the environment, such as layout, way finding, signage and storage, which increase efficacy, safety, reduce errors and improve the patient experience.

Other aspects of the environment which are important but often neglected are how it smells and sounds. The smell in a healthcare facility has in the past been associated with the quality of care (Wilks 1991), and in Chapter 10, Hugo Sax suggests that scent can affect health worker behaviours, including adherence to hand hygiene protocols. There is also evidence that the use of pleasant aromas or playing music can reduce anxiety (Graham et al. 2003; Drahota et al. 2012).

16.5 JOB SATISFACTION AND PERFORMANCE

Though job satisfaction and performance may be influenced by monetary rewards and management, the provision of a good physical working environment also affects satisfaction and performance (Newsham et al. 2009). Lambrou et al. (2010) found that difficult working conditions along with low pay were disincentives for healthcare workers. An optimal workplace environment in which employees feel safe, secure and supported improves performance and job satisfaction (Dharmanegara et al. 2016). There is also evidence that the built environment of the workplace is an important factor in creating and mitigating workplace stress (Vischer 2007b).

Shawn Achor (2011) argues that happy workers perform better and are less likely to take off sick days, leave or burn out. It may be expected that staff who enjoy coming to work and have good experiences are more likely to be compliant with expectations of practice, including infection control.

Many of us encounter people who complain that IPC compliance is made difficult by the environment they work in. Whilst some make heroic efforts to achieve best practice, others may struggle. Houghton et al. (2020) found that a lack of isolation facilities and space, overcrowding, access to hand hygiene facilities and the flow of infectious patients were key factors in ensuring staff adherence to IPC guidance. These factors are all related to the built environment and the infrastructure of the organisation. These may be barriers to optimal working practices and cause dissatisfaction. Other barriers to compliance identified included the lack of showering facilities for healthcare workers and spare capacity to clean and prepare rooms for new admissions.

The flow of people, equipment, supplies and waste within healthcare facilities is also a significant issue in the prevention of contamination and transmission of infection and may require significant investment and planning. This may include separate entrances, corridors, staircases or elevators or allocated parts of the facility to ensure separation. However, the effect on the ergonomics of those working in the environment may make this difficult to achieve and sustain unless it is carefully planned and monitored.

Example: In one organisation, the operating theatre staff were told that they could no longer mix with other hospital staff or patients in the general restaurant/canteen unless they first showered and changed out of their scrubs. As it took 15 minutes of a 30-minute break to walk to and from the canteen, this was unpopular. At the request of the theatre team, the catering team provided a drinks and sandwich trolley which visited the theatres during the day. This service was subsequently stopped as so much of the waste from refreshments was discarded in and around the theatres, causing additional work. Subsequently a break area was created adjacent to the theatres with catering facilities and a regular food delivery service.

The working environment reflects the cultural values of the organisation and indicates how much the employer values the employee (Vischer 2007a). This should include the entire team and does not just apply to senior clinical and managerial staff. It is not unusual for domestic, security and maintenance staff in health care to be provided with working areas which are small, cluttered, badly lit and ventilated and with minimal access to changing facilities or rest areas (Jeanes et al. 2012). Staff who are on relatively low wages doing nonclinical work require a similar quality and provision of facilities to clinical staff, managers and patients and visitors, and anything less will create dissatisfaction and affect motivation. Organisations which maintain an optimal working environment are more likely to have satisfied staff who help to maintain it (Hur & Nasar 2014).

16.6 PLANNING PROCESS

Planning a healthcare facility is complex and challenging. Experts, stakeholders (including local communities), finance departments, management teams and healthcare workers have differing experience, expertise and expectations. There may be changes during the planning process in, for example, the purpose and role of the facility, the funding available, the time scale, the size and the services required for enabling and supporting the build. Whilst many of us can envisage our own perfect healthcare and work environment, it is rare that we achieve it, and if we do, it is likely that others may not agree with all our choices or share our priorities, which are personal ideals and influenced by past experiences.

Participation in planning meetings is valuable in understanding the context and perspective of other people involved in this process. Other stakeholders will have their own expertise, terminology and priorities, some of which may be fundamental to the viability of the building. An example is fire safety, for which there are specific and mandatory requirements, specifications, and controls. Recognition of the safety and welfare concerns of stakeholders in the initial planning stage is important to the success of the planning project.

The applicable mandatory requirements and national IPC guidance are a significant starting point in planning facilities (Hignett & Lu 2009) if they exist but may require expert interpretation or adaptation. In some countries with limited IPC capacity, the role of international mandates and guidance is of relevance. The context and purpose of the facility is an important consideration. The design and infection controls required will vary considerably between, for example, a patient room in a hospice and an examination room in an emergency department.

It is also important to recognise that ICPs may not fully understand how different teams and specialities function within a space. Participation in functional space exercises where these teams work within a mock-up of space to ensure staff can function effectively help identify the constraints of the space and work undertaken (Hignett et al. 2010). Ensuring that maintenance and domestic teams are included in these exercises is essential to ensure that they can also function effectively.

Understanding the purpose and context of services and the needs of users is helpful in offering planning advice. There may not be one infection control answer which fits everyone. An example is the choice of floor covering, which may vary, for example, in a rapid treatment centre and a residential care home; in addition, this may vary from room to room depending on function, users' preferences and in response to innovations in flooring.

There may be a perceived tension between building to prevent and control infection and the provision of an environment that seeks to optimise and improve the quality of life for those being cared for (Anderson et al. 2020). There may be consequences to focusing on creating a perfect IPC environment. In the past, infection control has been perceived as rigid and dogmatic about what is possible or permitted, which may have been a barrier to the infection control team (ICT) participation in planning, building and renovation work. In addition, it may be perceived by the ICT as an added burden when the clinical workload is high, and this work may be allocated to someone with less experience or responsibilities and more time. These perceptions are being challenged and must continue to do so.

In the experience of the author, many (but not all) healthcare facilities are conceived, designed and built by people who never or no longer work there and who did not or will not experience the service delivered there. These absent participants have a major impact on what is finally delivered and the legacy it leaves behind. The rationale for some of the design and build decisions maybe lost through time, and those inheriting and working in the facility are dependent on the original building plans and notes to for example understand where the drains go, why there is no window or why there is no storage provision.

The limitations of organisational memory of the plan and build process is compounded by changes over time of those advising planners, the guidance available and the advice given. Unfortunately, infection control advice is rarely cut and dried, and there are frequently contradictory and changing views and opinions amongst ICPs. The guiding principles of the purpose and design of the build may be diluted or lost in the lengthy process of the build. This may be compounded by a frustration with some outdated mandatory building requirements which rarely change rapidly enough to reflect learning and experience (Hignett & Lu 2009).

In some instances, a dependence on professional planners and busy people who attend the requisite meetings can lead to a limited vision and a dependence on a minimal planning template, with little recognition of what else is possible. An industry standard based healthcare facility may be easy to replicate but ignores the context and needs of patients and staff (Price 2013).

Ironically in the UK and possibly elsewhere, the lengthy planning, financing and building process in health care can lead to the delivery of facilities which are already out of date by the time they are ready for use. It is therefore important to approach planning proactively by updating on the latest developments, visiting other facilities and seeking feedback from other users and colleagues. Significant change in health care is inevitable and an awareness of potential future requirements in infection prevention and control is valuable in supporting the planning process.

An integrative thinking approach (Martin & Austen 1999) enables the ICP to take advantage of the opportunities available in considering current issues and future developments. Examples include integrating smart building and nano technology, priming the environment to improve hand hygiene (King et al. 2016) and the use of olfactory conditioning to prompt behaviour change (Dmitrenko et al. 2018).

Feasibility and sustainability are also important considerations. This may vary, for example, in a temporary structure such as field hospitals or pop-up clinics and an established acute hospital in a well-resourced area. Sometimes ICTs need to be pragmatic and temper expectations, such as in times of disaster, war or pandemic in acceptance of what is "good enough."

The IPC perspective and planning advice should be rational, reasonable and compassionate. Effective healthcare facility planning is not a competition and requires compromises and teamwork.

16.7 PLANNING TERMINOLOGY

It is essential that IPC is involved and understands what is being planned as early as possible as the financial decisions are often made prior to the plans being drawn up, and every modification may incur added expense (Taylor et al. 2014). IPC advice, risks and opportunities will inevitably compete with other priorities for funds, location, functionality, developments.

Unless you are familiar with architectural terms and formats used, the process can be daunting. The language and terminology can be learnt, various technological formats are available and experience of the process makes it easier, but there may be pressures to respond rapidly and not to delay the planning process. This may be a steep learning curve.

In the UK the terms used in planning healthcare facilities often reflect historic titles and expectations of health care. Examples of terms which persist include "side rooms," "sluice," "clinical room," "clean utility," "dirty utility," many of which do not reflect their modern form and function. Consequently, the purpose of some areas may be ill defined, and new terms are needed to reflect use and risks of the healthcare environment. In Chapter 11 Kilpatrick et al. examine IPC language further.

16.8 POST-OCCUPANCY EVALUATION (POE)

The process of post-occupancy evaluation of facilities focuses on the perceptions and experiences of the built environment of the users after the facility has been in use for some time. The aim is to use feedback and objective evaluation of the area following a period of occupation to learn what works, what doesn't and what needs to be changed or fixed (Vischer 2002). The ICT contribution is valuable to this process as it can influence future planning, resource and design decisions.

Renovations or new builds based on planning assumptions about the purpose and usage of the facility may lead to unintended consequences. Examples include unused hand wash sinks in corridors, which are effectively a dead leg and therefore hazardous; doors which are frequently broken or left wedged open because of frequency of use or opening the wrong way and insufficient storage space.

Sometimes changes in purpose, function and usage are not foreseeable, and the provision is inadequate for what is required. Examples include a shift to more rigorous or corrosive cleaning and disinfection methods of the environment, which affects the integrity and durability of surfaces, or inadequate lift provision for the transfer of highly infectious patients.

POE is helpful in comparing how the facility was planned and how it is used. Two examples from an acute hospital include the following:

- Where do staff review notes and results or order tests and discuss cases? Is it the small, crowded office which is partly filled with spare mattresses or the reception area?
- Where do the relatives of visitors go to the toilet? Is it the designated toilets on the ground floor when their relative is on the fifteenth floor, or do they use a toilet designed for patients?

The IPC contribution to POE may include, for example, the ability to safely isolate when there is no clear line of sight, and extra staff are required to observe the area. The disruption of services related to outbreaks or incidents of preventable infection often has a financial implication for the organisation and may be a useful contribution or justification for change.

16.9 CONCLUSION

The built environment contributes to the risks and controls of infection in healthcare delivery. The involvement of ICTs in planning, refurbishment, building and maintenance is required to ensure that risks of infection to patients, staff and visitors are recognised, avoided, minimised and controlled.

Facilities which enhance the staff, patient and visitor experience contribute to a safe and supportive environment, which has significant benefits, including increased job satisfaction and positive patient outcomes, including reducing the risk of infection transmission.

It may be difficult to provide an environment which meets the needs of all users, and sometimes the available resource and capacity result in considerable compromise. Despite these constraints, consideration of the views, preferences, and experiences of users in healthcare buildings is a valuable opportunity to continuously improve what is provided. The Infection control implications of introducing innovative approaches to healthcare facilities and delivery require flexibility from IPC professions.

16.10 REFLECTIVE QUESTIONS

1. Do you take the context of care and preferences of patients into consideration when you or your team advise on the surfaces and finishes of new builds or renovations?
2. Have you participated in a post-occupancy evaluation in which you consider how the built environment has contributed to the transmission of infection?
3. Have you had the experience of being a visitor or patient in a healthcare facility? If so, what were your main observations about that built environment?
4. Has patient feedback about their experiences of the facilities you work in influenced your perception of the care delivered?

16.11 REFERENCES

Achor S. *The happiness advantage: The seven principles of positive psychology that fuel success and performance at work.* Random House. 2011.
Anderson DC, Grey T, Kennelly S, O'Neill D. Nursing home design and COVID-19: Balancing infection control, quality of life, and resilience. *Journal of the American Medical Directors Association.* 2020;21:1519–1524.
Brehm JW, Cohen AR. *Explorations in cognitive dissonance.* John Wiley & Sons Inc. 1962.

Browall M, Koinberg I, Falk H, Wijk H. Patients' experience of important factors in the healthcare environment in oncology care. *International Journal of Qualitative Studies on Health and Well-Being.* 2013;8(1):20870.

Burnett E, Lee K, Rushmer R, Ellis M, Noble M, Davey P. Healthcare-associated infection and the patient experience: A qualitative study using patient interviews. *Journal of Hospital Infection.* 2010;74:42–47.

Chen SI, Skillen DL. Promoting personal safety of building service workers: Issues and challenges. *Aaohn Journal.* 2006;54:262–269.

Dancer SJ. Controlling hospital-acquired infection: Focus on the role of the environment and new technologies for decontamination. *Clinical Microbiology Reviews.* 2014;27:665–690.

Dancer SJ. Infection control 'undercover': A patient experience. *Journal of Hospital Infection.* 2012;80:189–191.

Dharmanegara IB, Sitiari NW, Wirayudha ID. Job competency and work environment: The effect on job satisfaction and job performance among SMEs workers. *IOSR Journal of Business and Management.* 2016;18:19–26.

Dmitrenko D, Maggioni E, Obrist M. I smell trouble: Using multiple scents to convey driving-relevant information. *Proceedings of the 20th ACM International Conference on Multimodal Interaction.* 2018:234–238.

Douglas CH, Douglas MR. Patient-centred improvements in health-care built environments: Perspectives and design indicators. *Health Expectations.* 2005;8:264–276.

Drahota A, Ward D, Mackenzie H, Stores R, Higgins B, Gal D, Dean TP. Sensory environment on health-related outcomes of hospital patients. *Cochrane Database of Systematic Reviews.* 2012;3.

Edvardsson D, Sandman PO, Rasmussen B. Swedish language person-centred climate questionnaire–patient version: Construction and psychometric evaluation. *Journal of Advanced Nursing.* 2008;63:302–309.

Graham PH, Browne L, Cox H, Graham J. Inhalation aromatherapy during radiotherapy: Results of a placebo-controlled double-blind randomized trial. *Journal of Clinical Oncology.* 2003;21:2372–2376.

Hignett S, Lu J. An investigation of the use of health building notes by UK healthcare building designers. *Applied Ergonomics.* 2009;40:608–616.

Hignett S, Lu J, Fray M. Two case studies using mock-ups for planning adult and neonatal intensive care facilities. *Journal of Healthcare Engineering.* 2010;1:399–414.

Houghton C, Meskell P, Delaney H, Smalle M, Glenton C, Booth A, Chan XH, Devane D, Biesty LM. Barriers and facilitators to healthcare workers' adherence with infection prevention and control (IPC) guidelines for respiratory infectious diseases: A rapid qualitative evidence synthesis. *Cochrane Database of Systematic Reviews.* 2020;4.

Huisman ER, Morales E, van Hoof J, Kort HS. Healing environment: A review of the impact of physical environmental factors on users. *Building and Environment.* 2012;58:70–80.

Hur M, Nasar JL. Physical upkeep, perceived upkeep, fear of crime and neighborhood satisfaction. *Journal of Environmental Psychology.* 2014;38:186–194.

Jeanes A, Coen PG, Drey NS, Gould DJ. The development of hand hygiene compliance imperatives in an emergency department. *American Journal of Infection Control.* 2018;46:441–447.

Jeanes A, Hall TJ, Coen PG, Odunaike A, Hickok SS, Gant VA. Motivation and job satisfaction of cleaning staff in the NHS: A pilot study. *Journal of Infection Prevention.* 2012;13:55–64.

Jussim L. Self-fulfilling prophecies: A theoretical and integrative review. *Psychological Review.* 1986;93:429–445.

Kim M, Oh S. Assimilating to hierarchical culture: A grounded theory study on communication among clinical nurses. *PLoS One.* 2016;11:e0156305.

King D, Vlaev I, Everett-Thomas R, Fitzpatrick M, Darzi A, Birnbach DJ. "Priming" hand hygiene compliance in clinical environments. *Health Psychology.* 2016;35:96.

Lambrou P, Kontodimopoulos N, Niakas D. Motivation and job satisfaction among medical and nursing staff in a Cyprus public general hospital. *Human Resources for Health.* 2010;8:1–9.

Maben J, Griffiths P, Penfold C, Simon M, Anderson JE, Robert G, Pizzo E, Hughes J, Murrells T, Barlow J. One size fits all? Mixed methods evaluation of the impact of 100% single-room accommodation on staff and patient experience, safety and costs. *BMJ Quality & Safety.* 2016;25:241–256.

Martin R, Austen H. The art of integrative thinking. *Rotman Management.* 1999;12:4–9.

Newsham G, Brand J, Donnelly C, Veitch J, Aries M, Charles K. Linking indoor environment conditions to job satisfaction: A field study. *Building Research & Information.* 2009;37:129–147.

O'connell NH, Humphreys H. Intensive care unit design and environmental factors in the acquisition of infection. *Journal of Hospital Infection.* 2000;45:255–262.

Olmsted RN. Prevention by design: Construction and renovation of health care facilities for patient safety and infection prevention. *Infectious Disease Clinics of North America.* 2016;30:713–728.

Persky AM, Robinson JD. Moving from novice to expertise and its implications for instruction. *American Journal of Pharmaceutical Education.* 2017;81:72–80.

Price AD, Lu J. Impact of hospital space standardization on patient health and safety. *Architectural Engineering and Design Management.* 2013;9:49–61.

Simons DJ, Chabris CF. Gorillas in our midst: Sustained inattentional blindness for dynamic events. *Perception.* 1999;28:1059–1074.

Stockley JM, Constantine CE, Orr KE. Association of medical microbiologists' new hospital developments project group. Building new hospitals: A UK infection control perspective. *Journal of Hospital Infection.* 2006;62:285–299.

Suleyman G, Alangaden G, Bardossy AC. The role of environmental contamination in the transmission of nosocomial pathogens and healthcare-associated infections. *Current Infectious Disease Reports.* 2018;20:1–1.

Tanja-Dijkstra K, Pieterse ME. The psychological effects of the physical healthcare environment on healthcare personnel. *Cochrane Database of Systematic Reviews.* 2011;(1). Art. No.: CD006210. DOI: 10.1002/14651858.CD006210.pub3. Accessed 15 December 2021.

Taylor E, Hignett S, Joseph A. The environment of safe care: Considering building design as one facet of safety. *Proceedings of the International Symposium on Human Factors and Ergonomics in Health Care.* 2014 June;3(1):123–127. Los Angeles, CA: SAGE Publications.

Ulrich RS. How design impacts wellness. *The Healthcare Forum Journal.* 1992;35:20–25.

Ulrich RS, Zimring C, Zhu X, DuBose J, Seo HB, Choi YS, Quan X, Joseph A. A review of the research literature on evidence-based healthcare design. *HERD: Health Environments Research & Design Journal.* 2008;1:61–125.

Vischer J. Post-occupancy evaluation: A multifaceted tool for building improvement. *Learning from Out Buildings: A State-of-the-Practice Summary of Post-Occupancy Evaluation.* 2002;29:23–34.

Vischer JC. The concept of workplace performance and its value to managers. *California Management Review.* 2007a;49:62–79.

Vischer JC. The effects of the physical environment on job performance: Towards a theoretical model of workspace stress. *Stress and health: Journal of the International Society for the Investigation of Stress.* 2007b;23:175–184.

Wakefield E. Is your graduate nurse suffering from transition shock? *Journal of Perioperative Nursing.* 2018;31:47–50.

Wilks J. *Carbolic and leeches.* Hyperion Books. 1991.

Musings on Philosophy and Infection Prevention and Control

17

Julie Storr

Contents

I don't immediately see the philosophical significance of microbes . . . microbes just personally strike me as incredibly boring critters.

(anon)

DOI: 10.1201/9781003379393-20

17.1 INTRODUCTION

Based on the current and historical focus of infection prevention and control (IPC) guidance and publications, it is no surprise that those who work across all levels of health care tend to associate IPC with the technical rather than the social. Indeed, based on a lifetime of interactions with health workers across numerous settings, I am confident that were a word-association game played with the average healthcare worker, the words likely alighted upon would include germs, a long list of specific infections, microbiology, hand hygiene and most definitely personal protective equipment (PPE)—the latter now synonymous with IPC. Other words might include epidemiology, outbreaks, isolation, antibiotics and monitoring or surveillance. Words with more of a leaning towards branches of philosophy would be less forthcoming, although perhaps "ethics" might arise if people start to think about outbreak control and the related human experience. This is of little surprise. The overt link between IPC and philosophy does appear to be underexplored, and the literature on IPC *per se* and philosophy is not abundant. Infectious disease (ID) outbreaks is one area where matters of moral philosophy (ethics) and anthropology have been widely addressed, including within international guidance (WHO 2016a), but IPC is most certainly not ID.

There is a relationship between philosophy and anthropology which is described nicely in a paper by Khan and Tantray (2018). However, although both concern the study of human beings, they are different disciplines, as outlined in the definitions presented in Box 17.1. This chapter's main focus is philosophy, although it starts with an acknowledgement of the pioneering work of Macqueen on anthropological aspects of IPC. It aims to stimulate the reader to think beyond the status quo and consider what might be learned by focusing equally on social and technical sciences. It then starts to explore the philosophy of IPC beyond moral philosophy.

BOX 17.1   DEFINITION OF KEY TERMS USED IN THIS CHAPTER

Anthropology—the study of humankind, in particular the comparative study of human societies and cultures and their development.

Ethics—also referred to as moral philosophy, is concerned with the moral principles that govern a person's behaviour or the conducting of an activity. It is the branch of knowledge that deals with moral principles. Schools of ethics in Western philosophy can be divided into three sorts. The first draws on the work of Aristotle and holds that virtues such as justice, charity and generosity are dispositions to act in ways that benefit both the person possessing them and that person's society. The second, defended by Kant, makes the concept of duty central to morality. Humans are bound from a knowledge of their duty as rational beings to obey the categorical imperative to respect other rational beings. Thirdly, utilitarianism asserts that the guiding principle of conduct should be the greatest happiness or benefit of the greatest number.

Philosophy—the study of the fundamental nature of knowledge, reality and existence.

Primordial soup—a solution rich in organic compounds, in the primitive oceans of the earth from which life is thought to have originated.

Sentient—ability to sense or feel things.

Utilitarianism—the doctrine that actions are right if they are useful or for the benefit of a majority.

The New Oxford English Dictionary (2001)

17.2 IPC AND SOCIAL SCIENCES

This chapter is driven by a personal interest in the title's subject matter, and as a segue into this, I recall a presentation by a colleague—a former chair of the Infection Prevention Society, Sue Macqueen, on her work on anthropology (1995). This stood out at the time as unique, and it made me realise that there were important considerations related to what we do in IPC beyond the status quo. Her work is nicely summarised in a review that sought to remind IPC practitioners of the present, how Macqueen stimulated the IPC world to consider the biomedical cultural norms and influences that impact behaviour and implementation of IPC practices (Storr & Kilpatrick 2015). At that time, Macqueen introduced a new language, one that included reference not only to germ theory but also notions of dirt, symbolism, purity and ritualistic behaviour. In a parallel field, this was also the focus of much of the work of the late, self-proclaimed "disgustologist" Val Curtis and colleagues at the London School of Hygiene and Tropical Medicine, albeit mainly in a non-healthcare context (Curtis 2011). Two leaders, leading the way by stimulating practitioners to embrace social science thinking in their efforts to tackle infection and IDs. Kilpatrick explores the issue of language and IPC in detail in Chapter 11. Macqueen highlighted the powerful force of biomedicines' health message with regard to germ control that tended to overlook the cultural aspects in which it is practised and her work remains relevant to this day.

Social science thinking in IPC is increasingly being used, particularly with the growing appreciation that successful implementation of IPC interventions requires an understanding of behaviour change theories (Birgand et al. 2015), and those developing competency frameworks for IPC practitioners now recognise the need to embrace behaviour change theories in their efforts to implement guidance (WHO 2020). The social sciences therefore have much to offer in understanding why IPC remains a problem not yet solved in the twenty-first century. And so to philosophy and IPC, it will come as little surprise that this has not featured widely in the literature, but there is an interesting paper that summarises some key philosophical considerations, albeit largely related to matters of ethics (Bryan et al. 2007). Bryan et al. reflect on virtue ethics, which stresses the need to consider not only rules and outcomes but also the character of the individual(s) involved and communitarianism, which places special focus on community values and the common good. They aim to familiarize infection preventionists with some of the general frameworks associated with ethical dilemmas. The ethics of IPC will not be addressed here, a review of human rights, ethics and the impact of IPC measures on the psychosocial wellbeing of people can be found in Chapter 2 of our previous book (Storr 2016). In addition, although not the focus of this chapter, it is important to acknowledge that there is an ethical dimension of many IPC-related matters, including randomised controlled trials, genome sequencing and even the auditing of hand hygiene compliance (Meng et al. 2021).

17.3 THE PHILOSOPHY OF MICROBIOLOGY

The book *Philosophy of Microbiology* by Maureen O'Malley (O'Malley 2014) is a fascinating read for anyone interested in probing the connectivity between these two disciplines. Towards the start of the book, O'Malley recounts a communication between herself and a philosopher which throws up an interesting perspective:

> I don't immediately see the philosophical significance of microbes. . . . Microbes just personally strike me as incredibly boring critters. . . . They're not the sort of thing that I yearn to understand, despite their acknowledged biological significance. Lots of things are biologically significant but are not philosophically significant. . . . They're just too small!
>
> (Anon 2014)

A useful review of the book is provided by Clarke (2015), who challenges a number of the claims of O'Malley while reflecting on the issues raised and is summarised in Box 17.2.

BOX 17.2   SELECTED SUMMARY OF CLARKE'S
REVIEW OF *PHILOSOPHY OF MICROBIOLOGY*

The book makes the case that microbes have a major contribution to the philosophy of biology. It starts by reminding the reader that "microbes are the most important, diverse and ancient life forms on our planet." It postulates that the science of microbiology is the science of most significant living entities and their influence on the rest of life. The book attempts to persuade philosophers of these claims and explore how standard philosophical concepts may be rethought. The author gives a careful analysis of the sense in which microbes can model macrobes, emphasising that microbes are not simpler versions of macrobes, rather exemplars of many features that are general to all life. The conclusion collects some heterogeneous thoughts about microbial conservation, including questioning what should be saved from extinction (whales and pandas, or ammonia oxidisers?), origins of life research and the aims of philosophy of science. Together, these are intended to persuade the reader that any person concerned with trying to understand life ought to take microbes as central and foundational to all their investigations. However, O'Malley's claim, "Microbes are superior to macrobes, for philosophical purposes at least," is hard to justify. At whose expense ought the greater attention to microbes be given . . . insects? Plants? Biochemistry? "In her privileging of microbes over macrobes, it's almost as if O'Malley misses the point that we humans are macrobes, that we eat macrobes and keep them as our pets. For that matter her conclusion "keep microbes in mind!" is one that I can unhesitatingly endorse."

17.4 LOOKING AT IPC THROUGH A PHILOSOPHICAL LENS

A fundamental assumption that IPC has a purpose and a value and that IPC interventions centred on the pursuit of microbes as the enemy is justified from a moral perspective that draws on public health ethics and utilitarianism. Microbes are the problem, and IPC is the solution. And so international guidelines present the evidence on what needs to happen, both at a national level and in individual healthcare institutions, to ameliorate the problem and protect people from harm. International Health Regulations (WHO 2016b) exist that position IPC as a major force for global health and security, a key part of the prevention of outbreaks of highly transmissible infection. Within this context, IPC contributes to the prevention of global epidemics and pandemics (WHO 2015) and helps save lives. The moral case for action, in which we spend most of our days and focus most of our energy in IPC on trying to eradicate microorganisms in health care, in the pursuit of the wellbeing and survival of the human race, appears to be extremely compelling albeit it is important to acknowledge that this whole issue of utilitarianisms is fraught with dilemmas (Kirkwood 2009).

On a personal level, I have encountered a small number of situations that made me think a little more deeply about these matters. Here I will share a number of *triggers* that stimulated some early considerations that touch on the philosophy of IPC, some of which develop in congruence with the work of O'Malley. I acknowledge, these may appear somewhat extreme—this is deliberate since the aim is to push our thinking to consider things not usually considered.

17.4.1 Trigger 1: Is It Okay to Wipe Out an Entire Life Form to Protect Humans?

The seeds for this chapter were planted a number of years ago through the curious musings of myself and a couple of colleagues, each involved to varying degrees nationally and internationally in programmes that aimed to increase levels of hand hygiene by healthcare workers. A significant part of the strategies employed in these programmes involved promoting the use of alcohol-based hand sanitisers at the point of care. This "system change" was one novel element of a multimodal behaviour change strategy (WHO 2009). Theoretical discussions ensued around whether any studies or academic writings existed addressing the philosophical aspects of these strategies that have as their essence the annihilation of a life form. We pondered whether the issue of the moral value or worth of microbes or viruses had ever been explored but pretty soon arrived at a brick wall. The suffering and devastation caused by some microbes, paired with the fact that they are not plausibly a sentient life form, leads any consideration of the philosophical and even the ethical aspects of how we treat them down a blind alley, in our humble opinion. This is a rather simplistic summary of matters that involve many complex theories, ones that I as a non-philosopher cannot even begin to touch upon. The moral arguments around the worth or significance of microbes and other non-human animals is for others to explore and analyse, and this is touched upon a little later by authors with relevant credentials. Our bottom-line thinking was that the quest to eradicate microbes from the hands of health workers confers monumental benefits in terms of health and the prevention of infection—so from a utilitarian perspective, there could be said to be no case to answer for. And yet I would suggest that on one level there could be something potentially uncomfortable when considering the obliteration of our microbial companions that warranted further thought. The discussion certainly sparked a curiosity in exploring the extent to which philosophy has been addressed across wider issues of IPC.

17.4.2   Trigger 2: "I Don't Want All Those Dead Creatures on My Hand!" (Nurse, National Children's Hospital Costa Rica)

While involved in pilot testing the implementation of WHO's Guidelines on Hand Hygiene in Health Care in Costa Rica (Allegranzi et al. 2013), I was presented for the first and only time with an interesting piece of feedback that aligns with some of the emerging themes of this chapter. The backdrop to this story is the publication of a seminal paper (Pittet et al. 2000) which acted as the catalyst for the multimodal strategy mentioned earlier. The hand sanitisers work by killing microbes, being both germicidal—excellent at killing Gram-positive and Gram-negative vegetative bacteria and also effective at killing some enveloped (lipophilic) viruses (WHO 2009). The point-of-care placement was critical to support the necessary health worker behaviour change and widespread adoption of WHO's multimodal improvement strategy and has reportedly saved many lives (Crouzet 2014). However, after presenting the evidence and attempting to onboard colleagues to pilot test the approach in Costa Rica, I was somewhat surprised to learn via my translator that one of the nurses had reservations, stating, "*I don't want all those dead creatures on my hand!*" This prompted further feedback from others stating that they too were not comfortable with the thought that these hand sanitisers killed the germs but didn't remove them physically; the latter is achieved when washing hands at a sink with running water. Everyone including myself suddenly stared at their hands for what seemed like an eternity—all imagining millions of dead microbes piled high. Needless to say, the situation was resolved, and the strategy eventually adopted. The analogy between "creatures" and "microbes" is not an appropriate one. Costa Rica was one of the most successful of the pilot sites. Despite this, the perspective of the Costa Rican nurse certainly made me think about matters of microbial life and death in a slightly different way.

17.4.3 Trigger 3: Is Sentience the Ultimate Counter-Argument to the Moral Worth of Microbes?

Let me end with a hypothetical case. We travel back in time 3.5 billion years to the estimated period when Earth started to be inhabited by what is thought to be its first life forms—microorganisms, the seeds of which originated in what Darwin termed "primordial soup" (Marshall 2020). If this theory, one of many on the origins of life on Earth is correct, then it is on the existence of the chemical compounds in the soup—the precursors to unicellular organisms—that the future of mankind and our planet depends. The rudimentary organisms that evolved from the soup are not sentient beings, but they *are* the precursor to you and me—our ancestors, so to speak. They are surely a necessary link in the causal chain of the development of life on Earth. Imagine an alien presence landing on Earth for a fleeting moment having travelled the universe in a space machine, a sophisticated and advanced life form. Consider now that this extraterrestrial visitor destroys these early organisms, which have similarities to microbes, because they seem insignificant and lacking in sentience. Had this occurred, the sentient, living, breathing, sagacious humans of the twenty-first century most likely would never have existed.

All this led me to ponder a number of questions. First, are all microbes bad? It's clear that they are not—the widespread consumption of probiotics is a case in point. Given that some microbes are harmless and even beneficial, are there any issues relating to our efforts to eliminate from existence some microbes and preserve others? What influences our decisions? The next question is—are all viruses bad? The answer to this is not so clear. Mietzsch and Agbandje-McKenna (2017) state that if non-virologists were to be asked about viruses, the word "good" would be unlikely to arise. Indeed, they go on to say that most people associate instead, words such as "disease," "infection" and harm, influenced by media reports of infectious diseases such as HIV, Ebola and now COVID-19. In their paper "The Good That Viruses Do," these authors highlight how some viruses can be used to target cancer cells or help to deliver vaccines. So in conclusion—it's complicated!

17.5 VACCINATION AND ITS PHILOSOPHICAL IMPLICATIONS

Many readers will either have been involved in the delivery of vaccination programmes or studied this as part of their IPC and public health courses. Smallpox, a devastating disease that caused millions of deaths, was the target of a global eradication campaign, and this was successfully achieved in 1980, the only infectious disease to achieve this distinction (Nelson & Masters Williams 2014). However, some authors, including the microbiologist Bernard Dixon (1976), raised ethical issues associated with the drive to eradicate smallpox. He posed challenging questions on the justifications used to argue for the conservation of some species while pursuing the eradication of others. Dixon also introduced guilt into the fray, pondering why mankind feels guilt at the pending extinction of some large creatures while discounting the extinction of microbes, the arguments circling back to matters of sentience.

Immunization against a range of infectious diseases remains one of the most successful and cost-effective public health interventions (WHO Health Topics 2022). The Global Polio Eradication Initiative (GPEI) is working towards its promise of a polio-free world (Nelson & Masters Williams 2014). It is hard to understand how anyone might disagree with the eradication of these devastating IDs. However, resistance to immunization (described as vaccine hesitancy) reveals some interesting matters, including those relating to moral philosophy. A case study from the GPEI in Nigeria (Rubincam & Naysmith 2009) throws up a number of issues. Vaccination programmes require a compliant community for their success. In this real-world example, community leaders in Nigeria led a vaccination boycott, demanding improvements in access to food, other medicines and health care per se before they would accept the vaccination. This raised some key ethical issues relating to the impact of mandatory vaccination on human rights and autonomy. In addition, the socioeconomic situation of the target audience and their trust in the health system was also of relevance. Mandatory vaccinations threaten the autonomy of the target community. This case highlights the dichotomy between the basic human rights of a community to express autonomy and the motivation of the GPEI to meet its objectives. It is a stark reminder of the challenging moral landscape associated with attempts to eradicate a killer disease within a context where the recipients of the vaccination programme perceive their immediate threat to health to be from potential starvation rather than the virus.

17.6 PUSHING THE PHILOSOPHICAL THINKING EVEN FURTHER

Let us recap on the facts. First, IPC is concerned with eradicating some life forms off the face of the Earth, the use of bactericidal and viricidal hand sanitisers being one example. Second, some vaccination programmes are designed to consign their target microorganisms or viruses to history. Third, where IPC interventions fail to protect people, subsequent treatments such as antibiotics are designed to kill the offending microbes. Do any of these warrant a philosophical exploration, or is that pushing the bounds of sense? When considering the issues raised in Trigger 1 previously, we wondered whether any literature existed on the matter. A PubMed search reveals little of direct relevance in relation to IPC and philosophy. In addition to Dixon (1976), there are some papers on the controversial matter of the moral claims of microbes, including their rights and how they are treated by humans. These papers could be considered thought-provoking in the extreme, but they are relevant to the goals of IPC to some extent (Cockell 2011). Cockell highlights that in the 1970s a science fiction story explored the futuristic ramifications of full microbial rights, which could see a scenario in which household products such as bleach and deodorants were banned (Patrouch 1977). Cockell poses a crucial question around whether microbes possess any intrinsic value beyond their practical uses in such areas as food and drug production and the health of ecosystems. The paper by Cockell is of academic rather than practical interest, but it nonetheless raises some matters that are not conventionally considered within the specialty around the notion of respect and empathy towards other life forms, which microbes undoubtedly are, albeit not sentient ones. The author concludes and indeed clarifies that the needs of humans ultimately trump those of microbes—if this conclusion were not reached, he describes an absurd end point in which the 1970s fiction becomes reality.

REFLECTIVE EXERCISE

Before reading the conclusion, take a few moments to ponder on some of the issues raised in this chapter. Before you started reading the chapter had you ever reflected on any of these? Do you think there is any rationale for questioning the eradication of microbes from the world? What are your thoughts on vaccine hesitancy? Do you ever think there will be a book on IPC and philosophy, and if so, what might it address?

17.7 CONCLUSION

Much of what we do in IPC addresses moral philosophy. The multimodal hand hygiene improvement strategy is a behaviour change approach that aims to influence people to do something because of the moral imperative to protect vulnerable people from harm. But as was addressed in Chapter 8, some of the things that are undertaken in the name of IPC have consequences and can result in harms over and above that presented by the target microbe. This raises significant ethical concerns in itself. Microbes are the reason that IPC exists as a speciality. However, it is when microbes cause harm or have the potential to cause harm that they start to be seen as problematic rather than suggesting all microbes are bad. Undoubtedly many microbes are beneficial, but equally many, when they invade human cells, are killers. The philosophical imperative to tackle these problematic microbes is strong, and IPC programmes could be said to have an underlying philosophical imperative.

17.8 REFERENCES

Allegranzi B, Gayet-Ageron A, Damani N, Bengaly L, McLaws ML, Moro ML, Memish Z, Urroz O, Richet H, Storr J, Donaldson L, & Pittet D (2013, October) Global implementation of WHO's multimodal strategy for improvement of hand hygiene: A quasi-experimental study. *Lancet Infectious Diseases* 13(10):843–51.

Anon (2014) Anonymous philosopher of science, personal communication 2013. In Maureen A. O'Malley (ed.), *Philosophy of Microbiology*. Cambridge University Press.

Birgand G, Johansson A, Szilagyi E, & Lucet JC (2015) Overcoming the obstacles of implementing infection prevention and control guidelines. *Clinical Microbiology and Infection: The Official Publication of the European Society of Clinical Microbiology and Infectious Diseases* 21(12):1067–1071. https://doi.org/10.1016/j.cmi.2015.09.005

Bryan CS, Call TJ, & Elliott KC (2007, September) The ethics of infection control: Philosophical frameworks. *Infection Control & Hospital Epidemiology* 28(9):1077–84. doi: 10.1086/519863. Epub 6 July 2007. PMID: 17932830.

Clarke E (2015) Philosophy of microbiology, a review. *Notre Dame Philosophical Reviews*. https://ndpr.nd.edu/reviews/philosophy-of-microbiology/ accessed 31 January 2022.

Cockell CS (2011) Microbial rights? *EMBO Reports* 12(3):181. https://doi.org/10.1038/embor.2011.13.

Crouzet T (2014) *Clean Hands Save Lives*. L'age d'Homme, Thierry Crouzet and Thomas Clegg.

Curtis V (2011) Why disgust matters. *Philosophical Transactions of the Royal Society B: Biological Sciences* 366:3478–3490.

Dixon B (1976) Smallpox, imminent extinction and an unresolved dilemma. *New Scientist* 26:430–432.

Khan TR, & Tantray MA (2018) Philosophy and anthropology: A critical relation. *World Wide Journal of Multidisciplinary Research and Development* 4(5):230–234.

Kirkwood K (2009) In the name of the greater good? *Emerging Health Threats Journal* 2:e12. doi: 10.3134/ehtj.09.012.

Macqueen S (1995) Anthropology and germ theory. *The Journal of Hospital Infection* 30 Suppl:116–126. https://doi.org/10.1016/0195-6701(95)90012-8.

Marshall M (2020) Charles Darwin's hunch about early life was probably right. *BBC Future*, 11 November 2020. www.bbc.com/future/article/20201110-charles-darwin-early-life-theory.

Maureen AO (2014) *Philosophy of Microbiology*. Cambridge University Press.

Meng M, Seidlein AH, & Kugler C (2021, September) Hand hygiene monitoring technology: A descriptive study of ethics and acceptance in nursing. *Nursing Ethics* 15. doi: 10.1177/09697330211015351. Epub ahead of print. PMID: 34525855.

Mietzsch M, & Agbandje-McKenna M (2017) The good that viruses do. *Annual Review of Virology* 4:1, iii v. www.annualreviews.org/doi/full/10.1146/annurev-vi-04-071217-100011.

Nelson KE, & Masters Williams C (2014) *Infectious Disease Epidemiology: Theory and Practice*, Third Edition. Jones & Bartlett Learning.

Patrouch J (1977) Legal rights for germs. *Analog Science Fiction/Science Fact* XCVII(11):167–169.

Pearsall J, & Hanks P (2001) *The New Oxford English Dictionary*. Oxford University Press.

Pittet D, Hugonnet S, Harbarth S, Mourouga P, Sauvan V, Touveneau S, & Perneger TV (14 October 2000) Effectiveness of a hospital-wide programme to improve compliance with hand hygiene. *Infection Control Programme. Lancet* 356(9238):1307–1312.

Rubincam C, & Naysmith S (2009) Unexpected agency: Participation as a bargaining chip for the poor. *Health and Human Rights* 11:87–92.

Storr J (2016) Just infection prevention and control. In P. Elliott, J. Storr, & A. Jeanes (eds.), *Infection Prevention and Control: Perceptions and Perspectives*. Taylor and Francis.

Storr J, & Kilpatrick C (2015) *Journal Watch. Journal of Infection Prevention* 16(3):131–134. https://doi.org/10.1177/1757177415585594.

WHO (2015) *Ebola Response Phase 3: Framework for Achieving and Sustaining a Resilient Zero*. WHO.

WHO (2020) *Core Competencies for Infection Prevention and Control Professionals*. World Health Organization. https://apps.who.int/iris/handle/10665/335821 accessed 8 January 2022.

WHO Health Topics (2022) Immunization (web pages). www.who.int/news-room/facts-in-pictures/detail/immunization accessed 7 January 2022.

World Health Organization (2009) *WHO Guidelines on Hand Hygiene in Health Care*. World Health Organization. https://apps.who.int/iris/handle/10665/44102 accessed 4 February 2022.

World Health Organization (2016a) *Guidance for Managing Ethical Issues in Infectious Disease Outbreaks*. World Health Organization.

World Health Organization (2016b) *International Health Regulations (2005)*, 3rd Edition. World Health Organization.

Index

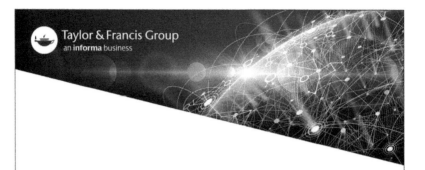

Milton Keynes UK
Ingram Content Group UK Ltd.
UKHW022040141024
449569UK00014B/667